HUMAN HELMINTHIASIS

Edited by **Luis Rodrigo**

Human Helminthiasis
http://dx.doi.org/10.5772/62673
Edited by Luis Rodrigo

Contributors

Hosni Khairy Salem, Mohamed S Abdeltawab Ali, Nala Seddik, Zilungile Mkhize-Kwitshana, Musawenkosi Mabaso, Rebecca Tadokera, Zhenhai Shen, Takafira Mduluza, Tawanda Chisango, Agness Nhidza, Amos Marume, Jose Barrios, Rodrigo Catharino, Estela De Oliveira Lima, Diogo Oliveira, Cibele Esteves, Tatiane Guerreiro, Carlos Melo

Published by InTech

Janeza Trdine 9, 51000 Rijeka, Croatia

Publishing Process Manager Dajana Pemac
Technical Editor SPi Global
Cover InTech Design team

First published February, 2017
Printed in Croatia
Legal deposit, Croatia: National and University Library in Zagreb

Additional hard copies can be obtained from orders@intechopen.com

Human Helminthiasis, Edited by Luis Rodrigo
p. cm.
Print ISBN 978-953-51-2953-0
Online ISBN 978-953-51-2954-7

For EU product safety concerns:
IN TECH d.o.o., Prolaz Marije Krucifikse Kozulić 3, 51000 Rijeka, Croatia,
info@intechopen.com or visit our website at intechopen.com.

Meet the editor

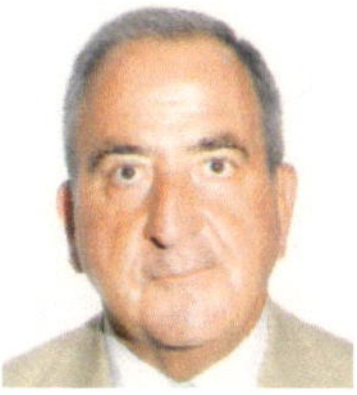

Dr. Luis Rodrigo, MD, is actually emeritus professor of Medicine at the University of Oviedo (Spain). He has been the chief of Gastroenterology Service at the University Hospital in Oviedo for 42 years. He obtained his PhD degree in 1975 and has developed a long teaching and research career during this time period. He is emeritus full professor of Medicine at the University of Oviedo, since 2014. He has published a total of 551 scientific papers, 270 written in English and the rest in Spanish. He has directed as main investigator in a total of 45 clinical trials. He has written around 35 chapters in books of several subjects and has been the editor of 13 books in his speciality.

Contents

Preface

Human helminthiasis is part of the neglected tropical diseases (NTDs) which are a diverse group of parasitic and bacterial diseases with distinct characteristics that thrive mainly among the poorest populations, hinder socioeconomic development, and cause substantial illness for more than one billion people globally. Seventeen NTDs have been specified by the World Health Organization (WHO). These NTDs impair physical and intellectual capacities of the affected persons, thereby perpetuating the cycle of poverty. Forty-seven countries in the African region are endemic to at least one NTD, and thirty-seven of them (79%) are coendemic to at least five of these diseases.

Zoonotic parasitic diseases are increasingly impacting human populations, due to the effects of globalization, urbanization, and climate change. The authors discuss those helminth diseases which are increasing in endemic areas and consider their geographical spread into new regions within the framework of globalization, urbanization, and climate change to determine the effect these variables have on disease incidence, transmission, and the associated challenges presented for public health initiatives, including control and elimination.

Although a considerable number of studies have been undertaken to date, it is still controversial as to whether or not coinfection with schistosomiasis increases the susceptibility to or the progression from hepatitis B virus (HBV) or hepatitis C virus (HCV) infection. One chapter analyzes this important topic. Greater use of the HBV vaccine is particularly advisable in endemic areas for schistosomiasis.

As genomic data for parasites are increasing, novel techniques for detection incorporating nucleotide sequences are receiving widespread attention. These sensitive, specific, and rapid detection methods are particularly important in the diagnosis of low-grade and early infections and may prove to have clinical significance. One chapter reviews the progress of nucleic acid detection in the diagnosis and prevention of schistosomiasis, including such aspects as the selection of target genes, and development and application of nucleic acid detection methods.

There is low-quality evidence that treating confirmed helminth infections in HIV-positive adults may have small, short-term favorable effects on markers of this disease progression. Further studies are required to confirm this finding. Current evidence suggests that deworming with anthelmintics is not harmful, and this is reassuring for the routine treatment of confirmed or suspected helminth infections in people living with HIV in coendemic areas. Further long-term studies are required to make confident conclusions regarding the impact of presumptively deworming all HIV-positive individuals, irrespective of helminth infection status, as the only long-term trial to date did not demonstrate a clear effect.

Also, there is an increased evidence on the role of helminth infections in modifying autoimmune and allergic diseases. These infections may have similar effect in other inflammatory processes, such as insulin resistance or the progression of atherosclerosis. Some studies have shown that helminth infections can be associated with improved metabolic outcomes. Understanding the mechanisms underlying this relationship could facilitate the development of novel strategies to prevent or delay the progression of type 2 diabetes mellitus.

Interventions that lead to reductions in soil-transmitted helminths (STHs) include chemotherapy with anthelmintic drugs and improvements in water, sanitation, and hygiene (WASH). In one of these chapters, the authors determine the evidence for optimal approaches for STH control. While multicomponent integrated control may be an effective approach to sustainably reduce STH transmission, there is a need for evidence to prove the feasibility of this approach.

I want to thank all the authors for their clear and very important contributions, as well as the speed and efficiency in sending their chapters on time. My heartfelt gratitude also to all the excellent team members from the InTech team, especially to Ms. Dajana Pemac for her continuous support through all the editorial process.

Prof. Luis Rodrigo, MD
Emeritus Professor of Medicine
University of Oviedo
Oviedo, Spain

Section 1

Epidemiology

Chapter 1

World Wide Epidemiology of Helminths Infection

Mohamed S. Abdeltawabi, Nahla El Seddik and

Hosni K. Salem

Additional information is available at the end of the chapter

http://dx.doi.org/10.5772/67273

Abstract

Helminths (from the Greek Helmins, meaning worm) include three groups of parasitic worm, large multicellular organisms with complex tissues and organs. Helminths do not replicate within the human host except *Strongyloides stercoralis*. Prevalence is commonly combined with worm burden (intensity of infection), which is commonly measured by the number of eggs per gram (EPGs) of faeces for intestinal helminths and schistosomes. Based on EPGs and their association with morbidity, individuals are classified into categories of light, moderate and heavy infection by the WHO. In the case of soil-transmitted helminths, the WHO recommends use of both prevalence and intensity of infection to classify communities into transmission categories—category I (high), category II (medium), and category III (low). The neglected status of the helminthiasis should be addressed on community levels and globally all over the world.

Keywords: epidemiology, helminths, infection, trematodes, cestodes, nematodes

1. Introduction, key determinants underlying the epidemiology of helminths infections

Helminths are worm-like parasites so they are commonly known as parasitic worms. They are classified mainly according to the morphology of the different stages; egg, larval and adult stages externally and internally [1].

Sexually, helminths have hermaphroditic species such as tapeworms and flukes except blood flukes. There also bisexual species like roundworms, the most common group worldwide is nematodes [1].

There are main three categories of helminths: trematodes (flukes), cestodes (tapeworms) and nematodes (roundworms) [1].

Studying epidemiology of helminths is highly important because they have a wide geographical distribution in different regions especially in sub-Saharan Africa, South America, Central America, Middle East, the Caribbean and Asia [2].

In 1998, the WHO Collaborating Centre for the Epidemiology of Intestinal Parasites at University of Oxford and WHO launched Global Atlas of Helminth Infections (GAHI) which is an initiative aimed at collating the available survey data as both a database and graphical tool (www.thiswormyworld.org) [2].

Based on GAHI, data collected between 1998 and 2010, on prevalence of helminths infections. Some data were collected older than these dates if no available data for a particular country.

Some countries were excluded based on their socioeconomic levels. And also three countries were excluded according to the comprehensive control such as Mauritius, Maldives and Mayotte. Seven countries in Oceania had no data, so they were assigned mean prevalence based on the regional data. Also eight countries had no data were assigned mean prevalence based on data of neighbouring countries with similar eco-epidemiological situation such as Georgia, Iraq and Turkmenistan data from Iran; Algeria data from Morocco; Syria and Tunisia data from Turkey; PDR Korea from Jilin Sheng (A province in China); and Timor Leste from Indonesia [2, 3].

Table 1 shows the distribution-prevalence of different helminths all over the world.

Helminthiasis	**Region**
Ascariasis *Ascariasis lumbricoides* (roundworm)	Asia, Africa and Latin America
Trichuriasis *Trichuris trichiura* (whipworm)	Asia, Africa and Latin America
Hookworm *Necator americanus; Ancylostoma duodenale*	Asia, Africa and Latin America
Strongyloidiasis *Strongyloides stercoralis* (threadworm)	Asia, Africa and Latin America
LF *Wuchereria bancrofti; Brugia malayi*	India, Southeast Asia and sub-Saharan Africa
Onchocerciasis (river blindness) *Onchocerca volvulus*	Sub-Saharan Africa
Loiasis *Loa loa*	Sub-Saharan Africa
Dracunculiasis (guinea worm) *Dracunculus medinensis*	Sub-Saharan Africa
Schistosomiasis *Schistosoma haematobium*	Sub-Saharan Africa
Schistosoma mansoni	Sub-Saharan Africa and Eastern Brazil
Schistosoma japonicum (blood flukes)	China and Southeast Asia
Clonorchis sinensis (liver fluke)	Developing regions of East Asia
Opisthorchis viverrini (liver fluke)	Developing regions of East Asia
Paragonimus spp. (lung flukes)	Developing regions of East Asia
Fasciolopsis buski (intestinal fluke)	Developing regions of East Asia
Fasciola hepatica (intestinal fluke)	Developing regions of East Asia
Cysticercosis *Taenia solium* (pork tapeworm)	sub-Saharan Africa and Sub-Saharan Africa

Table 1. The prevalence of human helminthiasis.

http://dx.doi.org/10.5772/67273

2. Epidemiology of trematodes (flukes)

2.1. Fasciola

They are highly distributed worldwide, and their reservoir hosts are not the human.

There are four species of Fasciola:

- *Fasciola hepatica*: It is found all over the world even in countries with high socioeconomic levels such as the USA and Europe. The unwashed watercress which is contaminated by the excreta of sheep is the mode of infection by eating it. It mainly affects the liver.
- *Fasciola gigantica*: It is found in Africa, Eastern Asia and Hawaii. Eating raw vegetables contaminated by the excreta of cattle and some mammals is the mode of infection. It mainly affects the liver.
- *Fasciolopsis buski*: It is found with high distribution in Far East and Indian Subcontinent especially Taiwan, Thailand, India and Bangladesh. Eating unwashed vegetables contaminated by human excreta or excreta of some pig mammals is the mode of infection. It mainly affects the intestine.
- Echinostoma species: They are found in South East Asia like Philippines and also in Japan. The mode of infection is ingestion of fresh water snails containing metacercaria. They mainly affect the intestine [1, 4].

2.2. Paragonimus westermani

It is a lung fluke which is found in South America and Eastern Asia. Eating raw seafood is the mode of infection. It mainly affects the lung and presents there encapsulated [1, 4].

2.3. Schistosomes

They are blood-dwelling trematodes. They have separate sexes.

It is estimated that 250 million people infected with Schistosomiasis by its major types: mansoni, haematobium and japonicum, more than 90% of them are in sub-Saharan Africa.

Also 500 million or more people are exposed to infection. The mode of infection is penetration of skin by cercaria. They mainly affect liver, lung, intestine and bladder.

There are three major species of Schistosomes:

- *Schistosoma haematobium*: It is found in Africa, Middle East and India. It affects the urinary tract.
- *Schistosoma mansoni*: It is found Central and West Africa, Egypt, Brazil, the Arabian Peninsula, Surinam, Venezuela, Madagascar and the West Indies. It affects the intestine and the liver. Also the infection starts with Katayama fever.
- *Schistosoma japonicum*: It is found in China, Japan, Indonesia and the Philippines.

There are also another two species but they have the same symptoms like *Schistosoma mansoni*:

- *Schistosoma intercalatum*: It is found in Central and West Africa.
- *Schistosoma mekongi*: It is found in Mekong River basin in Southeast Asia [1, 4].
- **Figure 1** showing the current global distribution of schistosomiasis worldwide [5].

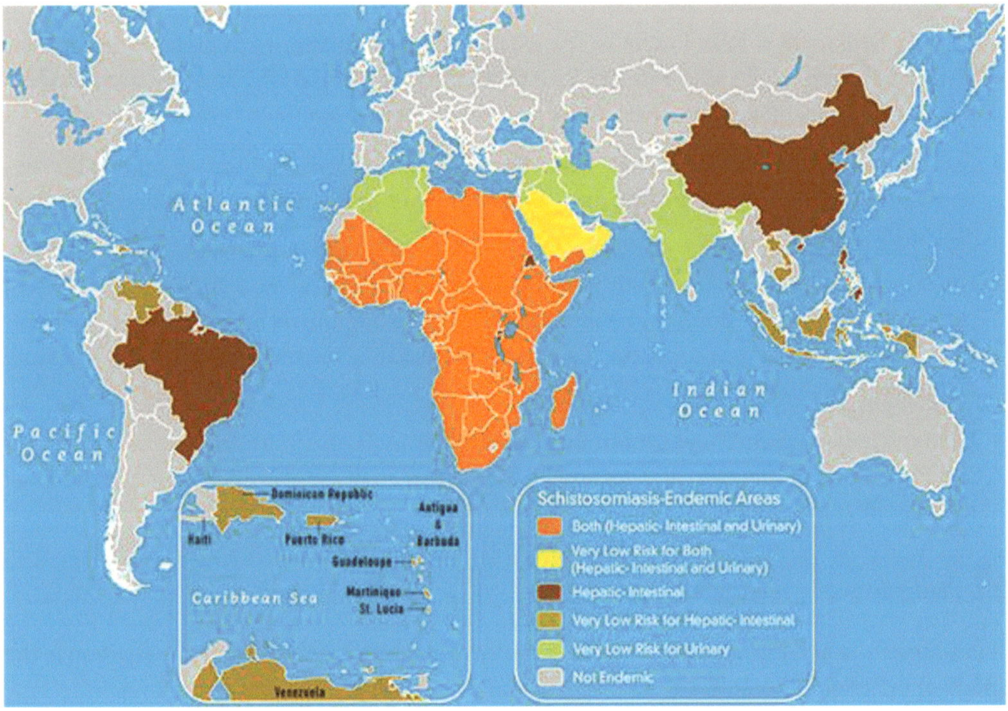

Figure 1. Map of the current global distribution of schistosomiasis. Source: US Centers for Disease Control and Prevention, <http://wwwnc.cdc.gov/travel/yellowbook/2012/chapter-3-infectious-diseases-related-to-travel/schistosomiasis#2696>) [5].

2.4. The oriental liver flukes

They are found in the Far East and Europe. The mode of infection is eating raw fish. They affect the liver.

There are three main species: *Clonorchis sinensis, Opisthorchis felineus* and *Opisthorchis viverrini* [4].

2.5. Heterophyes heterophyes

It is found in the Far East. The mode of infection is eating raw or pickled fish. It affects the small intestine [1].

2.6. Metagonimus yokogawai

It is found in the Far East. Eating raw or pickled fish is the mode of infection. It affects the small intestine [1].

http://dx.doi.org/10.5772/67273

Table 2 showing the diseases caused by flukes in the bile duct.

	Clonorchiasis	Opisthorchiasis	Fascioliasis
Parasite	*Clonorchis sinensis*	*Opisthorchis felineus*	*Fasciola hepatica*
Other mammalian hosts	Dogs, cats, pigs	Dogs, cats, foxes, pigs	Sheep, cattle
Mode of spread	Ova in faeces, water	As for *C. sinensis*	Ova in faeces on to wet pasture
1st intermediate host	Snails	Snails	Snails
2nd intermediate host	Freshwater fish	Freshwater fish	Encysts on vegetation
Geographical distribution	Far East, especially S. China	Far East, especially NE Thailand	Cosmopolitan, including UK
Pathology	*E. coli* cholangitis, abscesses, biliary carcinoma	As for *C. sinensis*	Toxaemia, cholangitis, eosinophilia
Symptoms	Often symptom-free, recurrent jaundice	As for *C. sinensis*	Unexplained fever, tender liver, may be ectopic, e.g. subcutaneous fluke
Diagnosis	Ova in stool or duodenal aspirate	As for *C. sinensis*	As for *C. sinensis*, also serology
Prevention	Cook fish	Cook fish	Avoid contaminated watercress
Treatment	Praziquantel 25 mg/kg 8-hourly for 2 days	As for *C. sinensis* but for 1 day only	Triclabendazole 10 mg/kg single dose; repeat treatment may be required

Table 2. The diseases caused by flukes in the bile duct.

3. Epidemiology of Cestode (tapeworms)

Table 3 shows the prevalence of human Cestodiases around the world.

Adult Cestodiases of Mankind		
Scientific name	**Site of infection**	**Distribution**
Diphyllobothrium latum	Small intestine	Argentina, Europe, Japan, Siberia, Great Lakes area, the USA
Taenia saginata	Small intestine	Everywhere
Taenia solium	Small intestine	Everywhere
Hymenolepis nana	Small intestine	Everywhere

Table 3. The prevalence of human Cestodiases (tapeworms).

3.1. Taenia species

They are the most common cestodes infect humans. They affect the intestine especially the duodenum.

There are two species of Taenia:

- *Taenia saginata*: It has a cosmopolitan distribution, but is more commonly found in developing countries due to poor socioeconomic levels and bad hygiene. The mode of infection is eating improperly cooked beef.
- *Taenia solium*: It is almost not present in the USA and Europe. The mode of infection is eating improperly cooked pork [6].

3.2. Hymenolepididae

They have a cosmopolitan distribution. The mode of infection by them is eating raw vegetables. They affect the small intestine.

There are four species of Hymenolepididae:

- *Hymenolepis nana*: It is thought to be the most common Cestode in the world. It affects children more than adults.
- *Hymenolepis diminuta*: It has a cosmopolitan distribution but it is found infrequently in humans.
- *Hymenolepis microstoma* and *Hymenolepis citelli*: They have been used extensively for studies on Cestodes [6].

3.3. Diphyllobothriidae

There are three species of Diphyllobothriidae:

- *Diphyllobothrium latum*: It has a cosmopolitan distribution but it is found mostly in countries bordering the Baltic Sea in Europe. The mode of infection is eating raw fish. It affects the small intestine.
- *Diphyllobothrium dendriticum* and *Diphyllobothrium ditremum* are mainly parasites of fish-eating mammals and birds [7].

3.4. Dipylidium caninum

Rarely, human is infected with *Dipylidium caninum*. Almost all reported cases are children. The mode of infection is eating raw vegetables. It affects the small intestine [7].

3.5. Larval cestodes

- *Echinococcus granulosus*: It is a larval stage of dog cestode. It causes Echinococcosis which is also known as hydatid disease due to development of hydatid cysts. These cysts can be located in the liver, the lung, the brain and the kidney. This disease is found commonly in Africa, the Middle East, South America and Australia. The mode of infection is eating raw vegetables.

- *Echinococcus multilocularis*: It is found in Europe, in the highlands like Switzerland, and also it is found in Alaska and Canada. The mode of infection is eating raw vegetables. Cysts are formed in the liver but they can later be located in the lung or the brain.
- *Multiceps multiceps*: It has a cosmopolitan distribution but mainly presents in the UK and the USA. The mode of infection is eating raw vegetables. Cysts are formed and located mainly in the spinal cord, the brain and the subcutaneous tissue [6].

4. Epidemiology of nematodes (roundworms)

Table 4 shows the prevalence of nematodes around the world.

Disease	Major etiologic agent	Global prevalence	Regions of highest prevalence
Soil-transmitted nematodes			
Ascariasis	*Ascariasis lumbricoides (roundworm)*	807 million	Developing regions of Asia, Africa, and Latin America
Trichuriasis	*Trichuris trichiura (whipworm)*	604 million	Developing regions of Asia, Africa, and Latin America
Hookworm	*Necator americanus, Ancylostoma duodenale*	576 million	Developing regions of Asia, Africa, and Latin America (especially areas of rural poverty)
Strongyloidiasis	*Strongyloides stercoralis (thread worm)*	30–100 million	Developing regions of Asia, Africa, and Latin America (especially areas of rural poverty)
Filarial nematodes			
LF	*Wuchereria bancrofti, Brugia malayi*	120 million	Developing regions of India, Southeast Asia, and sub-Saharan Africa
Onchocerciasis (river blindness)	*Onchocerca volvulus*	37 million	Sub-Saharan Africa
Loiasis	*Loa loa*	13 million	Sub-Saharan Africa
Dracunculiasis (guinea worm)	*Dracunculus medinensis*	0.01 million	Sub-Saharan Africa

Table 4. Global prevalence of nematodes (roundworms).

4.1. Ascaris lumbricoides

It is the largest intestinal nematodes found in humans. It has a cosmopolitan distribution, but it is more common in tropical and subtropical zones. The mode of infection is eating of raw vegetables. It affects the intestine and the lung [8].

4.2. Hookworm species

They are considered most destructive parasitic helminths infect human. Penetration of skin by Filariform larva is the mode of infection.

- *Necator americanus*: It is a New World hookworm. It is found in Far East, Asia, Africa, South America, and Oceania. It affects the small intestine.
- *Ancylostoma duodenale*: It is an Old World hookworm. It is found in the Middle East, North China, Europe, the Mediterranean countries, Africa, Asia and South America. It affects the small intestine.
- Cutaneous Larva migrans (*Ancylostoma braziliense* or *Ancylostoma caninum*): The mode of infection is contacting with hookworms larva of the dog or cat. They affect the skin [8].

Figure 2 showing the life cycle of Ancylostoma.

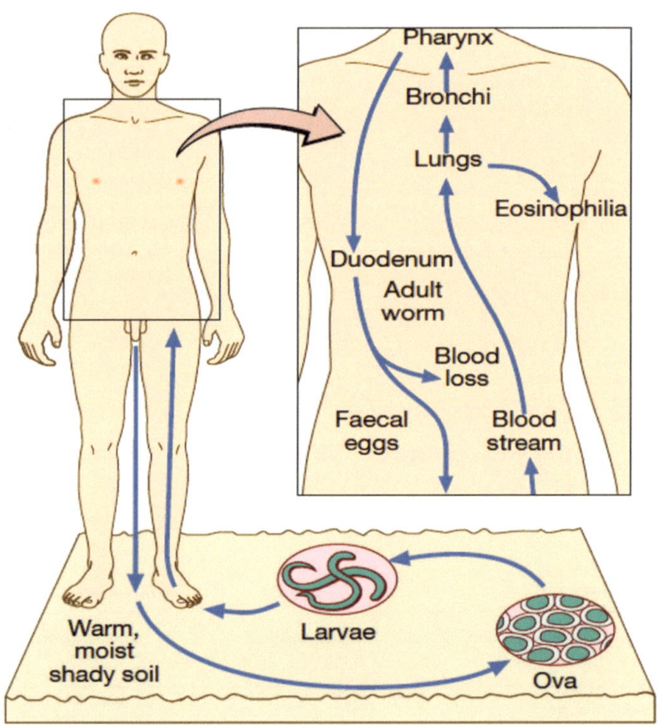

Figure 2. The life cycle of Ancylostoma.

4.3. Trichuris trichiura

It is known as the whipworm. Children are most commonly affected. It is found in tropical zones with poor sanitation. The mode of infection is eating raw vegetables. It affects the caecum and the upper part of the colon [1].

4.4. Strongyloides stercoralis

It is found in sub-tropical zones. Most of the 52 species of *Strongyloides* do not infect humans. *S stercoralis* is the most common human pathogen. Other species include *S myopotami* and *S procyonis*. These species have animal hosts and are thus responsible for zoonotic infections. Infections are initiated when exposed skin contacts contaminated soil. Autoinfection commonly occurs allowing infection to persist decades. Hyperinfection is typically triggered by drug-induced or disease-associated defects in cellular immunity, which allows a massive increase in parasite burden and dissemination to nearly all organ systems [9].

4.5. *Angiostrongylus* (Parastrongylus) *cantonensis*

It is also known as the rat nematodes. It is found in the Pacific areas, Central America and Cuba. The mode of infection is eating raw vegetables. It causes eosinophilic meningitis [1].

4.6. *Angiostrongylus* (Parastrongylus) *costaricensis*

It is found mainly in Costa Rica, but also some cases have been reported in Mexico, Central and South America. The mode of infection is eating raw vegetables. It affects the bowel wall [1].

4.7. Anisakiasis

It is found in Netherlands, North America, Canada, Chile, and the UK with the increasing spread of popularity of 'sushi'. There are two species causing human anisakiasis: *Anisakis simplex* and *Pseudoterranova osculatum*. The mode of infection is eating raw fish. It affects the intestine [1].

4.8. Gnathostoma spinigerum

It is found in Japan, China, the Far East and the Philippines; the mode of infection is eating raw freshwater fish. It affects the intestine and the cutaneous tissues [1].

4.9. Trichinella spiralis

It has a cosmopolitan distribution, and it is most commonly found in China and Europe. The mode of infection is eating raw pork. It affects the small intestine, the blood and the central nervous system.

According to the zones, temperature and infectivity, there are four types of it: *Trichinella spiralis* spiralis, *Trichinella spiralis* nelson, *Trichinella spiralis* nativa and *Trichinella spiralis* pseudospiralis [1].

4.10. Wuchereria bancrofti

It causes lymphatic filariasis. It is found in tropics and subtropics zones.

The mode of transmission is puncturing the skin by the vector, a mosquito.

Mosquitoes responsible for its transmission are *Culex quinquefasciatus, Anopheles gambiae* and *Anopheles funestus*.

It causes Lymphangitis commonly in the lower extremities and obstruction of the genital organs.

There are two strains of *Wuchereria bancrofti*:

- The nocturnal periodic strain which is found in Africa, India and the Far East.
- The sub-periodic strain which is found in the Pacific region [1].

4.11. Brugia malayi

It is found in South East Asia. There are two strains of *Brugia malayi*:

- The nocturnal periodic strain which is spread widely in Asia.
- The sub-periodic strain which is found in Malaysia, Indonesia and the Philippines.

The mode of transmission is puncturing the skin by the vector, Mansonia.

It affects the lymph vessels causing the same clinical picture of *Wuchereria bancrofti* [1].

4.12. Brugia timori

It is found in Indonesia. The mode of transmission is puncturing the skin by the vector, Mansonia. It affects the lymph vessels [1].

4.13. Loa loa

It is known as the African eye worm as it is found in West and Central Africa. The mode of transmission is puncturing the skin by the vector, Chrysops species.

It affects the skin causing Calabar swellings, which are inflammatory swellings resulting in a localized subcutaneous oedema [1].

4.14. Mansonella species

It is found in tropics and subtropics zones. The mode of transmission is puncturing the skin by the vector, Culicoides species. It affects the skin.

There are three species of Mansonella: *Mansonella perstans, Mansonella ozzardi* and *Mansonella streptocerca* [1, 8].

4.15. Onchocerca volvulus

It is found in central and West Africa. It is found also in South America.

The mode of transmission is puncturing the skin by the vector, Simulium (black flies), especially *Simulium damnosum*. It affects the skin and the eye [1, 8].

4.16. Dracunculus medinensis

It is found in Iran, India and Ghana in zones of little clean drinking water. The mode of transmission is ingestion of unclean water containing Cyclops.

It affects intestine and the lung [8].

4.17. Capillaria philippinensis

It is found in mainly Philippines and Thailand, but there were also some few unusual reports from Japan, Taiwan, Egypt and Iran. The source of infection is eating raw or improperly cooked fish. It affects the intestine [9–11].

4.18. Enterobius vermicularis

It has a cosmopolitan distribution. The modes of transmission are finger suckling, nail biting and eat raw vegetables.

It affects the small intestine [9–11].

According to a study performed in April 2008, the epidemiology of nematodes in developing regions of Asia, Africa, Latin and America as follows: *Ascaris lumbricoides* (807 millions), *Trichuris trichiura* (604 millions), hookworm (576 millions) and *Strongyloides stercoralis* (30–100 millions) [11].

Here are some examples of Nematodes' prevalence in different parts of the world:

a. Mazandaran province, northern Iran

Data analysis performed after examining unwashed raw vegetables for soil transmitted helminths showed below:

- The overall prevalence = 14.89%
- Contamination in warm seasons = 20.5%
- Contamination in cold seasons = 9.32%
- The prevalence of contamination is higher in leafy vegetables than root vegetables [12].
- The most common found species are as follows: *Ascaris lumbricoides, Trichuris trichiura,* hookworm, *Toxocara canis, Taenia solium* and *Hymenolepis nana* with prevalence: 3.36, 2.2, 2.9, 1.68, 0.9 and 2.2%, respectively.

b. Kampala, Uganda

Cross sectional survey in September and October 2013 applied on five groups of people:

- Workers maintaining wastewater facilities.
- Workers managing faecal sludge.
- Urban farmers.

- Slum dwellers at risk of flooding.
- Slum dwellers without work of flooding.
- They were tested using Kato-Katz stool sampling which showed:
- Highest prevalence in urban farmers = 75.9%
- Lowest prevalence in workers managing faecal sludge = 35.8%
- Hookworm is the predominant by 27.8%
- In urban farmers, the prevalence of Trichuris, Schistosoma mansoni and Ascaris was 15% and above [13].

c. Bungoma county, Western Kenya

Cross sectional study held in 2016 by examining cryopreserved stool samples of 796 persons with age ranges from 2 to 81 years revealed; prevalence of Ascaris lumbricoides (17%) and *Trichuris trichiura*, Ancylostoma and Strongyloides (less than 1.0%) [14].

d. Tezi Town, Puge county of Liangshan prefecture, Southwestern China

Cross sectional study from October 23 to November 3, 2014 showed prevalence of *Ascaris lumbricoides* (13.5%), *Trichuris trichiura* (30.6%) and both(7.1%) [15].

Mansonella ozzardi is a rare nematode but mainly present in The Americas from southern Mexico to northwestern Argentina with prevalence rate (0–46%) [16].

5. Future perspectives

There is being some changes in several countries due to the efforts to treat actively these parasites. Nevertheless, some negative circumstances such as wars, climate changes and poverty may influence in this growing problem.

The neglected status of the helminthiasis should be addressed on community levels and globally all over the world.

Author details

Mohamed S. Abdeltawabi, Nahla El Seddik and Hosni K. Salem*

*Address all correspondence to: Dr_hosni@kasralainy.edu.eg

Faculty of Medicine, Cairo University, Cairo, Egypt

References

[1] Castro GA, Baron S. editor. Medical Microbiology, 4th edition. University of Texas Medical Branch at Galveston, Galveston (TX); 1996. ISBN-10: 0-9631172-1-1.

[2] Pullan RL, Smith JL, Jasrasaria R, Brooker SJ .Global numbers of infection and disease burden of soil transmitted helminths infections in 2010. Parasit Vectors. 2014 Jan 21; 7:37. doi:10.1186/1756-3305-7-37

[3] Hotez PJ, Brindley PJ, Bethony JM, King CH, Pearce EJ, Jacobson J. Helminth infections: the great neglected tropical diseases. J Clin Invest. 2008 Apr 1; 118(4): 1311–1321. doi:10.1172/JCI34261. http://www.ncbi.nlm.nih.gov/pmc/articles/PMC2276811/

[4] Fürst T, Duthaler U, Sripa B, Utzinger J, Keiser J. Trematode infections: liver and lung flukes. Infect Dis Clin North Am. 2012 Jun; 26(2): 399–419. doi:10.1016/j.idc.2012.03.008

[5] David U Olveda, Yuesheng Li, Remigio M Olveda, Alfred K Lam, Thao N P Chau, Donald A Harn, Gail M Williams, Darren J Gray, Allen G P Ross. Bilharzia: pathology, diagnosis, management and control. Trop Med Surg. 2013 Aug 20; 1(4): 135. doi:10.4172/2329-9088.1000135

[6] Ammann RW, Eckert J. Cestodes. Echinococcus, Gastroenterol Clin North Am. 1996 Sep; 25(3): 655–89.

[7] Craig P, Ito A. Intestinal cestodes, Curr Opin Infect Dis. 2007 Oct; 20(5): 524–32.

[8] Walker MD, Zunt JR, Neuroparasitic infections: nematodes. Semin Neurol. 2005 Sep; 25(3): 252–61.

[9] Harhay MO, Horton J, Olliaro PL. Epidemiology and control of human gastrointestinal parasites in children. Expert Rev Anti Infect Ther. 2010 Feb; 8(2): 219–34. doi:10.1586/eri.09.119

[10] Walker MD, Zunt JR. Neuroparasitic infections: cestodes, trematodes, and protozoans. Semin Neurol. 2005 Sep; 25(3): 262–77.

[11] Jasmer DP, Goverse A, Smant G. Parasitic nematode interactions with mammals and plants. Annu Rev Phytopathol. 2003; 41: 245–70.

[12] Rostami A, Ebrahii Mm, Mehravar S, Fallah Omrani V, Fallahi S, Behniafar H. Contamination of commonly consumed raw vegetables with soil transmitted helminth eggs in Mazandaran province, northern Iran. Int J Food Microbiol. 2016.

[13] Fuhrimann S, Winkler MS, Kabatereine NB, Tukahebwa EM, Halage AA, Rutebemberwa E, et al. Risk of intestinal parasitic infections in people with different exposures to wastewater and fecal sludge in Kampala, Uganda: a cross-sectional study. PLoS Negl Trop Dis [Internet]. Public Library of Science; 2016 Mar 3 [cited 2016 Aug 26];10(3):e0004469. doi:10.1371/journal.pntd.0004469

[14] Easton AV, Oliveira RG, O'Connell EM, Kepha S, Mwandawiro CS, Njenga SM, et al. Multiparallel qPCR provides increased sensitivity and diagnostic breadth for gastrointestinal

parasites of humans: field-based inferences on the impact of mass deworming. Parasites & Vectors [Internet]. 2016; 9(1): 1–12. doi:10.1186/s13071-016-1314-y

[15] Xiao P-L, Zhou Y-B, Chen Y, Yang Y, Shi Y, Gao J-C, et al. Prevalence and risk factors of *Ascaris lumbricoides* (Linnaeus, 1758), *Trichuris trichiura* (Linnaeus, 1771) and HBV infections in Southwestern China: a community-based cross sectional study. Parasites & Vectors [Internet]. 2015; 8(1): 1–11. doi:10.1186/s13071-015-1279-2

[16] Lima NF, Veggiani Aybar CA, Dantur Juri MJ, Ferreira MU. *Mansonella ozzardi* : a neglected New World filarial nematode. Pathog Glob Health [Internet]. 2016; 110(3): 97–107. Available from: http://www.tandfonline.com/doi/full/10.1080/20477724.2016.1190544

Section 2

Diagnosis

Chapter 2

Mass Spectrometry and Metabolomics—New Approaches for Helminth Biochemical Studies

Estela O. Lima, Cibele Z. Esteves, Diogo N. Oliveira, Tatiane M. Guerreiro, Carlos F. O. R. Melo and Rodrigo R. Catharino

Additional information is available at the end of the chapter

http://dx.doi.org/10.5772/65040

Abstract

Metabolomics, the study of the endogenously synthesized small molecules repertoire (nonproteinaceous), is of great relevance for establishing a wide view of cell physiology at specific moments, linking metabolic profiles to phenotypes and genotypes. To better understand biological systems, such as helminths life cycle, helminthic infection, and host-parasite interaction, metabolomics studies are crucial. For that, mass spectrometry-based metabolomics is the most popular strategy. Nontargeted metabolomics allows researchers to profile entire metabolomes present in cells, tissues, biofluids, or even samples as complex as stools. Through different mass spectrometric techniques, it is possible to unveil chemical markers for helminths, such as *Schistosoma mansoni* (a trematode) and *Ascaris lumbricoides* (a nematode), in addition to study mechanisms of action for different drugs, which targets parasites. Therefore, mass spectrometry allows designing biochemical pathways that may clarify the processes of parasite life cycle, helminthic infection, and host-parasite interaction, providing targets to further interference for parasite control or even infection treatment.

Keywords: metabolomics, mass spectrometry, helminths, *Ascaris lumbricoides* , *Schistosoma mansoni*

1. Introduction

1.1. Metabolomics and mass spectrometry in biomedical research

The composition of the intracellular environment depends on harmonic and orchestrated synthesis and interaction of molecules that are essential for cellular survival and healthy life maintenance [1], and it is true for both eukaryotic and prokaryotic organisms. Eukaryotic cells present a higher degree of intricacy compared with prokaryotic cells because of the huge biochemical complexity they present [2]. Helminths represent a pluricellular eukaryotic group of worms that establish parasitic relationships with humans, which has been registered since ancient Greek writings [3]. Structurally, helminths are completely different from *Homo sapiens*, and it is assured that peculiar metabolic differences exist between these organisms. These differences enable understanding and studying helminth-human interaction, transmission routes, and life cycles through molecular studies, the cornerstone in all fields of biomedical research.

The search for faster, more accurate methodologies that describe the biochemical/pathophysiological status of an organism of interest has driven major efforts in biomedical research in the late years in order to meet the clinical needs for a health community [4]. Bioanalytical methodologies have then emerged as suitable choices for expeditious approaches that exhibit great resolution and sensitivity, thus generating the development of more accurate and precise methodologies. In instrumental bioanalysis, several compounds of interest can be measured and/or monitored depending on their molecular nature. As there is no "one-size-fits-all" approach, different molecular classes have demanded the creation of different analytical strategies in which both comprehensive and specific analyses can be performed. This, therefore, has elicited the development of the "omics" strategies, which were subdivided according to the needs of the researchers. For example, for large and bulky molecules such as proteins, a wide array of analytical methods compose what is called the proteomics approach, which is dedicated to study each and every aspect of proteins and their levels, interactions, and structure in biological systems [5]. The same rationale was then applied for other biological components, such as genes (genomics) [6], lipids (lipidomics) [7], and small molecules/ metabolites (metabolomics) [8].

Metabolomics can be understood in more detail as the systematic study of small, nonprotein, both endogenous and exogenous molecules, which represent the end of the entire biological chain started by gene expression (i.e., phenotype) [9]. Metabolomics studies usually measure compound classes such as lipids, nucleic acids, amino acids, and glycans, composing a useful biochemical platform for studying mechanisms of interactions, signalling synthetic pathways of systems and molecules under different metabolic conditions (e.g., diseases), providing specific molecules or molecular groups that characterize such conditions: the biomarkers. This assists in understanding, diagnosing, preventing, and predicting conditions, as well as helps assessing risks and benefits of pharmacological interventions [10].

Cell metabolism is one of the challenges that have been the driving force of metabolomics over the years [11]. The efforts on development were to obtain increasingly accurate and well-resolved methods, introducing more sophisticated and specific methods such as nuclear magnetic resonance (NMR) and mass spectrometry (MS) [12]. This made room for a number of improvements also in data processing and bioinformatics, where multivariate analyses and big data analytics found a whole new application in resolving and integrating complex biological matrices and systems [13], giving rise to the four main metabolomics strategies: metabolic profiling, the identification and quantification of known metabolites that are related to a specific number of metabolic pathways [14]; metabolic fingerprinting, which comprises fast-paced analysis to classify a determined sample during high-throughput screenings (positive/negative or disease/health) [15]; metabolic footprint, which analyses the extracellular metabolites (i.e., excretion/secretion products) of a given organism [16]; and targeted analysis, a series of quali-quantitative analyses of any given known metabolite in an orga-nism or a metabolic pathway [17].

The technical aspects of both NMR and MS place them both as the main tools for metabolomics studies, especially for their complementary nature. NMR is a spectroscopy-based technique that relies on the incidence of a magnetic field over the nuclei of atoms with nonzero spin counts, such as ^{1}H, ^{13}C, and ^{15}N, thus providing accurate structural and quantitative information of the metabolic profile under study [18]. There are several advantages associated with the use of NMR as an analytical tool for metabolomics; as it is not a destructive analysis, i.e., it is possible to recover the sample after the analysis, which is useful especially for target analyses. Moreover, NMR requires little sample preparation and shows great reproducibility, two desirable features for bioanalyses [19]. In contrast, some disadvantages hamper the wide distribution of NMR as a routine approach; the high costs associated with instrument maintenance and the need for relatively high amounts of the analyte usually turn down NMR as a high-throughput choice, which finds its best use as a research tool.

Mass spectrometry, on the other hand, despite being sample-destructive, shows great potential for routine analyses. MS-based bioanalytical systems show superior performance in detection and quantification limits, easily reaching a working range of nano to picomoles [20]. Relying on a basic structure of ionization source-mass analyser, MS brings a wide array of combinations of both, which comprehends virtually any type of sample for metabolomics studies [21], in addition to the possibility of coupling with chromatographic approaches such as gas chromatography (GC) and high-performance liquid chromatography (HPLC) [22]. Moreover, structural elucidation strategies with MS are diverse and can be suited according to the needs and to the instrument available, either with mass accuracy on high-resolution instruments or with fragmentation profile (MS/MS) in standard devices—or even a combination of the two [23]. These factors contributed to the popularization of MS among researchers and clinical experts and have, therefore, provided the basis for great development in this area.

Hence, this chapter will provide a comprehensive overview on the application of metabolomics analysis and strategies developed for the analyses of helminths, with a particular focus on MS, reinforcing the great importance of these organisms for general public health. The main aim is to address recent analytical chemistry methodologies, challenges to overcome and promising results, expanding possibilities at helminthiasis research, and thus contributing with advances in the area.

2. Biochemical characterization of helminthic parasites

2.1. *Schistosoma mansoni* biochemical characterization

S. mansoni metabolomics studies are conducted to improve the knowledge of disease pathology, to evaluate the behaviour and infectivity of different strains, to elucidate mechanisms of action, and to evaluate the efficacy of available drugs in addiction to discover biomarkers that can be applied as diagnostic and drug targets [24].

The main analytical metabolomics approaches are MS and NMR [25], and both of them allow performing target or untargeted analysis, which are mostly focused on two classes of metabo-lites: lipids and oligosaccharides. In case of living organisms, such as parasites, lipids are necessary for cell-cell signalling, for protection from host immunity, for maintenance of integrity and parasite structure during the life cycle and are also involved in the mechanisms of sexual development, egg production, and cercaria penetration [26–28]. Concerning oligosaccharides, these molecules are precursors of glycoconjugates such as glycoproteins and glycolipids that are mainly involved in development of innate and adaptive immune response in the host, parasite survival, and the chronic infection establishment [29, 30]. Lipids as well glycans may change as long as the parasite develops, thus it is crucial to understand metabolomics patterns according to the different lifecycle stages for each parasite studied.

2.1.1. Metabolomics approach for S. mansoni lifecycle stages

2.1.1.1. Mature and immature eggs

The main class of lipids present at *S. mansoni* eggs is glycosphingolipids [31], which are involved in interactions with the different affected organs, such as gut, lungs, or liver, facilitating its passage through the tissues [32]. Glycosphingolipids are also reported to be associated with egg's high immunogenicity and pathogenicity in different strains [33]. For example, the granuloma formation occurs by the reaction of host immune response mediated by parasite glycoconjugates; therefore, the greater abundance of glucosylceramides (GlcCer) in one strain compared to another, the higher pathogenicity [32, 34]. The same study using high-resolution mass spectrometry (HRMS) showed that phosphatidic acid (PA), phosphatidylserine (PS), phosphatidylethanolamine (PE), triacylglycerol (TG), and diacylglycerol (DG) are involved in the differentiation of *S. mansoni* strains [34]. In respect to maturation, immature and mature eggs present also been differentiated using Matrix-Assisted Laser Desorption/ Ionization—Time of Flight Mass Spectrometry (MALDI-TOF-MS). This research showed that immature eggs have a common N-glycan profile and are formed predominantly of nonspecific oligomanoses, while mature eggs have highly complex and fucosylated N-glycans [30]. Therefore, lipid molecules in eggs show differences according to maturation phases and diverge between distinct strains.

2.1.1.2. *Miracidium*

This is about a free-living and motile form that penetrates in *Biomphalaria sp.* snails, the intermediate host of the *S. masoni* lifecycle. Different strains were analyzed by HRMS, and the results showed the possibility to differentiate two strains of miracidium by identifying different lipids: triacylglycerol (TG), phosphatidylserine (PS), phosphatidic acid (PA), phosphatidylinositol-ceramide (PI-Cer), and dodecanoid acid (DA). The most interesting lipid among them is the last compound, reported to be responsible for facilitating the penetration of miracidium in snails [27]. Considering glycolipid studies through MALDI-TOF-MS analysis, miracidium glycolipids have been almost devoid of LeX- or LN-motifs, what is coherent with previous data that showed snail infection is apparently independent of LeX-motifs, but LDN-motifs are fairly present in miracidium and snail. Observing that the parasite presented the same spectra compared to the intermediate host, miracidium appear to develop a snail-compatible glycosylation pattern [30]. These molecular studies show lipid variability and/or similarity among different lifecycle stages, opening opportunities to better understand interactions between parasite and host/intermediate host or to interfere at metabolic pathways, as long as we know where and how [30, 35].

2.1.1.3. *Cercaria*

Cercaria, the final larval stage of *S. mansoni* lifecycle, produces secretions that facilitate skin penetration. These fluids are reported to be weak immunogenic and composed of glucoproteins and glycolipids. Mass spectrometry approaches demonstrate the predominance of ceramides-linked glucose and/or galactose with fucose and xylose cores at cercaria secretions [30, 33, 36]. Another study also determined the cercaria differentiation between two *S. mansoni* strains by HRMS. The lipids TG, DG, PE, PA, and phosphatidylglycerol (PG) were reported to be responsible for this discrimination [27].

2.1.1.4. *Adults*

The tegument surface structure of *S. mansoni* adult worms is crucial for parasite survival and modulation of host immune response. This structure is syncytial and is covered by two closely apposed lipid bilayers, one of them is an inner plasma membrane and the other an outer membranocalyx complex [28, 37]. Mass spectrometry studies conducted with tegument and whole worm demonstrate an enrichment of the phosphatidylcholine (PC) and PS of tegumental compositions, but this phenomena does not occur with PE and PI, which presents the same composition for the two worm fractions. The tegumental membranes are also enriched with lysophospholipids, mainly lyso-PS and lyso-PE containing eicosanoic acid (20:1) [28].

As regards glycans, their composition dramatically changes during the development stages. Comparing with early life-stages, adult worms present smaller ratio between complex type-glycans and oligomannosidic glycans and the antigenic core composed by xylose is undetectable [30].

Mass spectrometry imaging (MSI) enables the study of spatial distribution of biomarkers. Ferreira and co-workers (2014) used MALDI-MSI to image two different *S. mansoni* strains.

Figure 1 shows the sum of all ions obtained by the imaging analysis where it is possible to detect both male and female worms' bodies. The spectra obtained from the single worms were compared with the pair and enabled the election of specific ions for male and female worms [34].

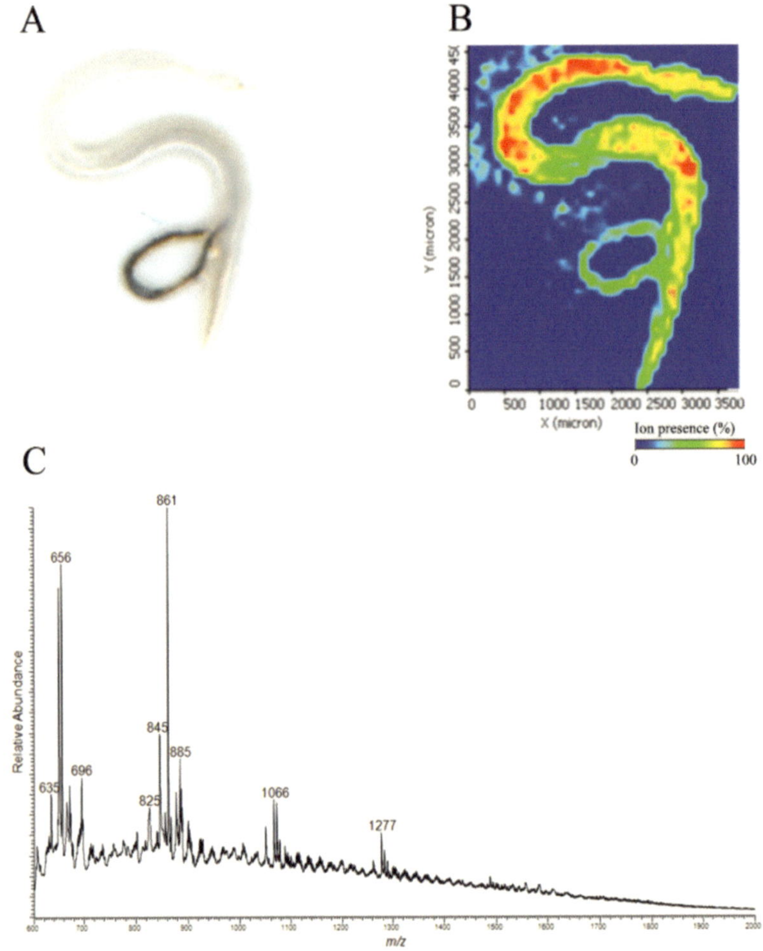

Figure 1. Representative fingerprinting of *Schistosoma mansoni* adult couple worms. The imaging represents a sum of all ions within mass range 600–2000 m/z. (A) Picture of worms analyzed. Gynaecophoric channel in male's body (clear) holding female's body (dark). (B) Worms' image generated by MALDI-MSI instrument. Illustrative picture of fingerprinting analysis. (C) Representative fingerprinting (total ion current) spectra. Positive ion mode.

The same study determined the ions responsible for the differentiation of male and female worms of two different strains and their localization in a worm body. The fingerprint of each worm was submitted to Principal Component Analysis (PCA), and the groups of strains are discriminated, enabling the selection of chemical markers for each group. New MS/MS imaging was performed and the distribution of the parental ions selected by PCA can be seen in **Figures 2** and **3**.

http://dx.doi.org/10.5772/65040

Figure 2 shows the male and female image of BH strain obtained by MALDI-MSI analysis. Female worm presents the predominance of PC (823, 665 and 761 m/z) and PG (764 m/z) distributed to reproductive and digestive systems. Male worm presents diacylcglycerol (DAG) (635 and 651 m/z) in ventral sucker and gynaecophoric channel, triacylglycerol (TAG) (846 and 886 m/z) in ventral sucker and reproductive system, phosphatidic acid (PA) (675 m/z) in ventral sucker and gynaecophoric channel, PI (862 m/z) in reproductive and digestive systems and ventral sucker, and finally, PC (887 m/z) in reproductive system and ventral sucker.

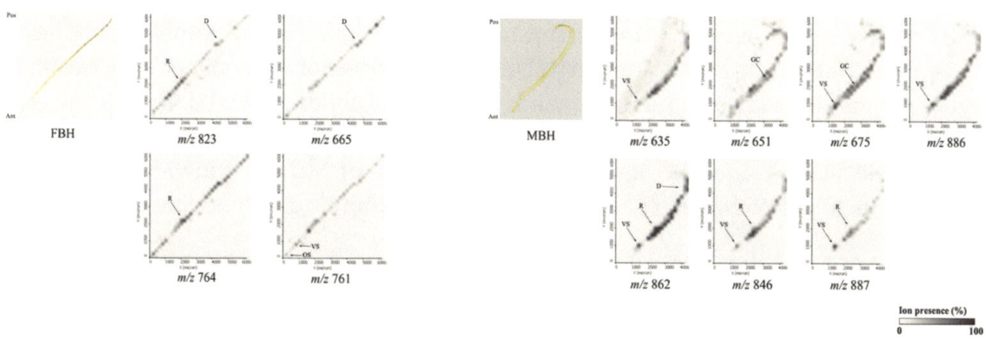

Figure 2. Adult worms generated by MS, selected using each of the parent ions in MS/MS mode. Images were acquired as one run for each m/z. Female and male BH strain (FBH and MBH, respectively). Pos, posterior portion; Ant, anterior portion; R, reproductive system; D, digestive system; VS, ventral sucker; OS, oral sucker; and GC, gynaecophoric channel.

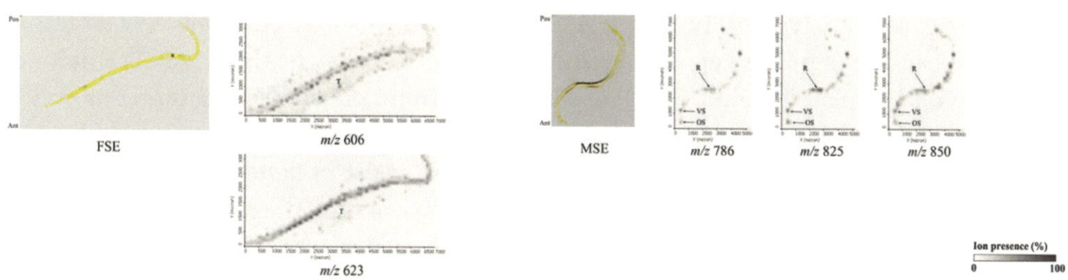

Figure 3. Adult worm images generated by MS, selected using each of the parent ions in MS/MS mode. Images were acquired as one run for each m/z. Female and male SE strain (FSE and MSE, respectively). Pos, posterior portion; Ant, anterior portion; R, reproductive system; VS, ventral sucker; and OS, oral sucker.

Figure 3 shows male and female image of SE strain obtained by MALDI-MSI analysis. Female worm presents the predominance of PI (623 m/z) and DAG (606 m/z) distributed mainly in tegument while male worm presents TAG (786 and 850 m/z) and PC (825 m/z) in ventral and oral suckers and reproductive system.

Ferreira and coworkers (2014) demonstrate that it is possible to determine spatial distribution of biomarkers for parasites and also show that more studies are necessary to understand the function of each chemical markers according to the organs they are located, searching for its influence through pathogenicity of different strains. Furthermore, a new platform of study putting together metabolomic and mass spectrometry techniques was proposed and was named as Parasitomics.

2.2. *Ascaris lumbricoides* and chemical markers at *moulting* process

According to Pullan and coworkers [38] and CDC [39], it is estimated that 800–1200 million people are infected with *Ascaris lumbricoides* worldwide and more than 60,000 deaths occur annually because of *Ascariasis* (spectrum of disease caused by *Ascaris lumbricoides* infection). World Health Organization has applied some strategies for disease burden control, such as deworming programmes [40]. In case of soil-transmitted helminthiasis, the main public health strategy is the mass drug administration (MDA), which consists of anthelmintic drug treatment regularly provided to risk population, mainly school-aged children [40, 41]. Despite the great efforts, approximately 30% of children are really receiving the anthelmintic treatment in the whole world [42]. Besides the absence of total coverage of MDA worldwide, there is still another issue to pay attention, the development of anthelmintic drug resistance [43–45].

Taking into account all of these issues cited above, beyond the disability-adjusted life years (DALYs) in consequence of morbidity and mortality indexes, it is necessary to better comprehend and to deal with helminthic parasites, such as *Ascaris lumbricoides*, in a different point of view. It is urgent to evaluate and discover different and better ways to control and eliminate it. Therefore, to outline strategies that are suitable for its life cycle could bring light to management of helminthiasis. Since part of the development of *A. lumbricoides* happens in the soil [46, 47], it is therefore reasonable to consider that breaking the life cycle during the phases in the environment would be a valuable attempt in containing the infection in endemic areas [48].

Molecular detailed analysis of the *diverse A. lumbricoides* forms may elucidate new targets for parasite control. Metabolic fingerprinting using mass spectrometry has been widely employed, targeting parasite-related metabolites [34, 49, 50]. The trend of establishing target molecules and linking them with important metabolic pathways in the parasite life cycle broadens the knowledge in the field, generating a platform that will assist in better knowledge on their biology, elucidation of survival mechanisms, pharmacodynamics, diagnostic methodologies, development of pharmaceutical products to eradicate these diseases, whether in soil or living hosts, etc. [50, 51].

Melo and coworkers aimed to characterize, in a simple way, the larval development stages of *A. lumbricoides* (the traditional human ascariasis agent) by metabolic fingerprinting using HRMS from stool samples [52]. The molecular elucidation in different life stages presents a huge potential for application in parasite infection control, breaking the life cycle and reducing infection and re-infection of exposed human beings, mainly at endemic zones.

From *Ascaris lumbricoides* specimens, it is possible to separate different development larval stages using optical microscopy. Melo's researchers group analyzed stool samples collected from school-aged children at Brazil. Nonembryonated and embryonated eggs, containing L1 and L3 larvae, could be separated from stool pool. L2 stage larvae were excluded from samples because it is an overlapping period between the end of L1 and the beginning of L3, what makes it difficult to identify and isolate. Considering the high sensitivity of mass spectrometer analyser, it was necessary to clean as much as possible this complex sample, what favors the real identification of significant molecules [52].

For molecular screening like this, starting from a complex sample, it is necessary to do a multivariate statistical analysis for correct identification of targets. For the present study, Principal Component Analysis (PCA) was chosen to statistically determine relevant groups of ions, what led to identification of the correspondent molecular biomarkers for each development stage under analysis. From the elected ions by PCA, it was possible to achieve the most suitable chemical markers through metabolome databases analysis, along with a good literature review. ESI-HRMS analysis of *Ascaris lumbricoides* specimens showed different spectral signals among the egg, L1 and L3, and PCA statistical analysis elected distinct chemical markers for each structure/larval stage.

2.2.1. Metabolomics approach for A. lumbricoides lifecycle stages

2.2.1.1. Eggs

Considering eggs analysis, it was possible to identify five biomarkers: hexadecenal (515 m/z), 21-Methyl-8Z-pentatriacontene (522 m/z), 3,7,11,15-Tetramethyl tetratriacontane (565 m/z), and two unsaturated fatty acids, corresponding to 537 m/z. The phospholipid hexadecenal may probably be a by-product of sphingosine-1-phosphate (S1P) degradation. Hexadecenal is associated with cytoskeleton reorganization, JNK-dependent apoptosis, and proliferation signalling pathways. Since the analyzed eggs were under embryogenesis, JNK pathway may favor cell proliferation and embryo development [53–55]. Taking into account that hexadecenal appears only in the mass spectra of eggs, it may be acting in signalling during embryonic development process according to weather conditions, food availability and population, among others [56].

Two other signals elected by PCA, 21-Methyl-8Z-pentatriacontene (522 m/z) and 3,7,11,15-Tetramethyl Tetratriacontane (565 m/z), correspond to signalling molecules in insects, although their function is not clear yet. There were still two unsaturated fatty acids elected for eggs (537 m/z) that, based at their carbon chain, it is supposed they have a role at preventing water loss, considering that fertilized eggs are constantly at high risk of dehydration in the soil [57, 58].

2.2.1.2. L1 moulting stage

Considering biomarkers statistically elected for L1, a total of four molecules were selected. One of them, 2-deoxyecdysone-22-phosphate (563 m/z), is a steroid hormone source found during insects embryogenesis. These steroid hormones, commonly called ecdysones, are associated with control of development in insects and nematodes, processes called moulting [59]. Taking into account that ecdysone synthesis depends on cholesterol [60], it is necessary for the nematode to absorb it. Therefore, it could explain the election of cholesteryl ester (CE) as a second biomarker at L1 stage [61, 62].

The lipid composition may vary according to environmental conditions and parasite life stage. Elected as L1 biomarker, cardiolipins are examples of molecules present at the inner mitochondrial membranes [63], whose constitution may vary to adapt to different aeration conditions. Considering that the development of *A. lumbricoides* occurs through different life stages with distinct air availability [64], it is coherent that oxidative stress conditions interfere with mitochondrial lipid composition. In addition to cardiolipins, sphingolipids (SPL) were one of the chemical markers elected at L1 stage. SPL is an important class of lipids and may be modified according to the cycle life stage, just similarly as it happens with insects' development [65].

2.2.1.3. L3 moulting stage

The last larval stage studied at Melo's work was L3, and one of the possible markers was Dimethylheptatriacontane. It is a signalling molecule involved with sexual communication between arthropods, better known as pheromone [66]. Considering nematodes and arthropods are closely related, some hypothesis were raised about its function at *A. lumbricoides* L3: (i) it could play the same role as in arthropods; (ii) to stimulate sexual differentiation during parasite development [67]; (iii) to act as a "messenger" during development according to environmental conditions [56]. Depending on the life stage, this *signalling* molecule may present more than one function, but the exact role of dimethylheptatriacontane at nematodes is still to be unveiled.

Considering all biomarkers elected for different lifecycle stages for *Ascaris lumbricoides*, it is possible to observe that there is a whole metabolic parasite world to discover and establish connections. Therefore, it is too important to keep looking for new biochemical pathways that explain parasite similarities, survival, development, host invasiveness, and immunogenicity. Only the entire knowledge will answer the unsolved questions and allow human interference to improve health conditions and social development.

3. Searching for drug targets at helminthiasis—Praziquantel and *Schistosoma mansoni* chemical targets

It is estimated that about 2 billion people in the world, especially the inhabitants of developing regions such as sub-Saharan Africa, East Africa, Asia, and the Americas are infected with one or more helminths, making parasitic diseases very expensive for public health [68–70]. The drugs used until now to treat these diseases are far from ideal, and many of them were introduced decades ago [71, 72]. Most of these drugs are related to serious adverse effects, which supports the low adherence to treatment by patients. Moreover, these drugs have limited efficacy and can have their activity paralyzed due to the phenomenon of drug resistance [72, 73]. The treatment of such parasitic diseases is mainly related to two factors: sanitation and health education, which when combined with the use of anthelmintic drugs promote the success of treatment and avoids occurrence of new cases [73, 74].

Ascariasis is a parasitic disease caused by infection with the nematode *Ascaris lumbricoides*, which is one of the soil-transmitted helminthiasis that head the list of the so-called "Neglected

Diseases" [69, 75]. This parasitic disease has been associated with intestinal pathology, respiratory symptoms, and malnutrition in children from endemic areas [76, 77]. The indicated treatment for Ascariasis is based at anti-helminthic drugs against *A. lumbricoides*, which have been found to be safe and effective. Single oral doses of Albendazole, Mebendazole, and Pyrantel pamoate have demonstrated high cure rates against this parasite [69].

Albendazole and Mebendazole are Benzimidazole-based compounds, which are the most widely used anthelmintics until now [75]. These medicines are known as antimicrotubule agents due to their therapeutic effect by relating with the capacity of binding to free β-tubulin. This attachment inhibits tubulin polymerization and disrupts microtubules, which loses structure and function, leading the organism to death [78, 79]. The selective toxicity of these agents results because Benzimidazoles bind parasite β-tubulin with much higher affinity than the mammalian protein [80]. However, there are evidences of drug resistance due to existence of cases where loss of efficacy has been reported after administration of a single dose [44, 81].

Schistosomiasis is also part of the list of "Neglected Diseases" and is responsible for infecting more than 200 million people in tropical and subtropical regions of the world, especially in sub-Saharan Africa [82, 83]. Introduced in the early 1980, Praziquantel (PZQ) is the drug of choice in the treatment of schistosomiasis. The detailed molecular mechanism of action of PZQ has not yet been fully explained, but it is related with tegumental damage and paralytic muscular contraction of parasites via influx of Ca^{2+} across the tegument [74, 84].

PZQ is a safe anthelmintic, but cases of drug resistance are already known, such as reported for ascariasis. The first field report came from a new and epidemic focus in northern Senegal [85]. Many infections that persisted after treatment and were not detected by the usual diagnostic methods (with eggs per gram below the detection limit of the coprological techniques) required repeated or very sensitive examinations [86, 87]. Thus, the recommended doses of medicine for schistosomiasis should be considered subcurative [88], and it is safe to assume that in schistosome populations, some individual parasites are tolerant to the drug, at least at the usual dosages [73].

The phenomenon of anthelmintic resistance is a genetic modification that can be defined as a state of insensitivity or decreased sensitivity to the effect of a determined drug concentration, conferring a number of parasites of a given population the capacity to survive the pharmacological effect of recommended therapeutic doses of an anthelmintic [75]. In veterinary practice, frequent treatment of closed populations has led to a serious problem of anthelmintic drug resistance, which is now largely irreversible [73]. Thus, it is urgently needed to search and develop sensitive tools for early detection and monitoring of drug resistance, as well as new anthelmintic evaluation of drug combinations for parasite control.

Drug discovery is an iterative process where different strategies can be applied. Usually, it can be divided into several distinct stages, starting with target identification and validation, proceeding to assay development and screening (whole cell or target molecular basis) and ending with hits identification. Thenceforward, it is necessary to synthesize and evaluate analogues to verify the structure-activity relationships and identify the elected hit; to optimize its structure, interactive medicinal chemistry is used, and finally, it is done on all preclinical development before the clinical evaluation [71].

Target-based drug discovery starts with the identification and elucidation of the function of a potential therapeutic drug target and understanding its role in the disease process. Drug targets are, basically, molecular structures that will undergo a specific interaction with chemicals (drugs), which are administered to treat or diagnose a disease. Most of the times, drug targets are enzymes or proteins involved in biological activity, which are produced by expression of active genes in a cell [70]. Furthermore, it is interesting to develop drugs whose targets include biochemical pathways, such as cellular physiological process or cell *signalling* molecules. For example, it has been reported as an inhibitor of programmed cell death pathway (apoptosis) to be a potential small molecule acting on a caspase to control schistosomiasis caused by *S. japonicum* [89]. Therefore, metabolic pathways can also be explored as therapeutic targets, where there should be a clear understanding of anthelmintics mechanisms of action operating in helminth parasites [70].

For exploratory studies as cited above, metabolomics is a very powerful tool to connect parasite metabolism and its interaction with the drug of choice. To better understand some of these mechanisms, chromatographic techniques combined with MS have been employed for chemical characterization of adult schistosomes and PZQ metabolites in the host [90, 91]. In a study from 2015, researchers used MS Imaging (MALDI-MSI) to better understand some of the mechanisms of interaction between PZQ and schistosomes. The researchers were able to characterize both sexes of *S. mansoni* adult worms (BH strain) treated with PZQ and identified the spatial distribution of chemical markers. In addition to tegumental damage, PZQ significantly changed the metabolic profile of both sexes of *S. mansoni* [49]. These data are supported by a recent work where tegumental damage of schistosomes under PZQ exposure was demonstrated through scanning electronic microscopy and optical microscopy [92]. These findings could be helpful for understanding possible targets and pathways of this anti-schistosomal drug and demonstrates the versatility and potential use of mass spectrometry-based metabolomics for identification of drug targets.

4. Conclusions

New tools are now available for biomedical research, and mass spectrometry techniques are among them. In "omics" research, huge opportunities are rising and enable to understand mechanistic basis for biological differences. For example, the absence of an enzyme in determined disease might be compared with healthy samples, unveiling significant molecular differences that clarify the mechanisms of action associated with a genetic failure. This new approach for biological systems allows the correlation between genotype and phenotype aspects, which is a complex process nowadays. Metabolomics studies are now giving the molecular profile of health or disease just like a "snapshot" of cell physiology. It is up to us scientists to establish the right and coherent correlations between metabolic patterns and biological alterations.

Although helminthiasis still consists of a neglected disease, concerning all the discussed topics, it is possible to keep looking for new strategies that help to control and treat these infections. The groups of molecules identified by metabolomics approaches, exemplified as MS, might be tested and correlated with the proposed hypothesis, and then it may be possible to finally understand the parasites metabolism. In this way, it will be possible to comprehend the mechanisms of all different lifecycle stages, expanding the field of action for parasite control. In addition, metabolomics can bring light to the designing of new therapeutic drugs, highly effective and specific, reducing collateral effects and drug resistance.

Therefore, mass spectrometry and metabolomics show huge potential as new tools to unveil metabolism of different biological systems, including helminths. The more scientists unveil about metabolism of parasites and parasite-host interactions, the greater the chances of improving public health aiming a better future.

Author details

Estela O. Lima, Cibele Z. Esteves, Diogo N. Oliveira, Tatiane M. Guerreiro, Carlos F. O. R. Melo and Rodrigo R. Catharino*

*Address all correspondence to: rrcatharino@gmail.com

Innovare Laboratory of Biomarkers, University of Campinas, Brazil

References

[1] Wilson DF. Regulation of cellular metabolism: programming and maintaining metabolic homeostasis. Journal of Applied Physiology (Bethesda, Md: 1985). 2013;115(11): 1583–8. Epub 2013/10/12.

[2] Doolittle WF. A paradigm gets shifty. Nature. 1998;392(6671):15–6.

[3] Cox FEG. History of human parasitology. Clinical Microbiology Reviews. 2002;15(4): 595–612.

[4] Hare DJ, New EJ. On the outside looking in: redefining the role of analytical chemistry in the biosciences. Chemical Communications. 2016;52(58):8918–34.

[5] Cox J, Mann M. Is proteomics the new genomics? Cell. 2007;130(3):395–8.

[6] Johnston DA, Blaxter ML, Degrave WM, Foster J, Ivens AC, Melville SE. Genomics and the biology of parasites. Bioessays. 1999;21(2):131–47.

[7] Wenk MR. Lipidomics of host–pathogen interactions. FEBS Letters. 2006;580(23): 5541–51.

[8] Kafsack BF, Llinás M. Eating at the table of another: metabolomics of host-parasite interactions. Cell Host & Microbe. 2010;7(2):90–9.

[9] Roessner U, Bowne J. What is metabolomics all about? Biotechniques. 2009;46(5):363.

[10] Weckwerth W. Metabolomics: an integral technique in systems biology. Bioanalysis. 2010;2(4):829–36.

[11] Patti GJ, Yanes O, Siuzdak G. Innovation: metabolomics: the apogee of the omics trilogy. Nature Reviews Molecular Cell Biology. 2012;13(4):263–9.

[12] Pan Z, Raftery D. Comparing and combining NMR spectroscopy and mass spectrometry in metabolomics. Analytical and Bioanalytical Chemistry. 2007;387(2):525–7.

[13] Katajamaa M, Orešič M. Data processing for mass spectrometry-based metabolomics. Journal of Chromatography A. 2007;1158(1):318–28.

[14] Harrigan GG, Goodacre R. Metabolic Profiling: Its Role in Biomarker Discovery and Gene Function Analysis. Springer Science & Business Media; Dordrecht, Netherlands. 2012.

[15] Ellis DI, Goodacre R. Metabolic fingerprinting in disease diagnosis: biomedical applications of infrared and Raman spectroscopy. Analyst. 2006;131(8):875–85.

[16] Kell DB, Brown M, Davey HM, Dunn WB, Spasic I, Oliver SG. Metabolic footprinting and systems biology: the medium is the message. Nature Reviews Microbiology. 2005;3(7):557–65.

[17] Weljie AM, Newton J, Mercier P, Carlson E, Slupsky CM. Targeted profiling: quantitative analysis of 1H NMR metabolomics data. Analytical Chemistry. 2006;78(13):4430–42.

[18] Barding Jr GA, Salditos R, Larive CK. Quantitative NMR for bioanalysis and metabolomics. Analytical and Bioanalytical Chemistry. 2012;404(4):1165–79.

[19] Pettegrew JW. NMR: Principles and Applications to Biomedical Research. Springer Science & Business Media; New York - USA. 2012.

[20] Han X, Gross RW. Structural determination of picomole amounts of phospholipids via electrospray ionization tandem mass spectrometry. Journal of the American Society for Mass Spectrometry. 1995;6(12):1202–10.

[21] Venter A, Nefliu M, Cooks RG. Ambient desorption ionization mass spectrometry. Trends in Analytical Chemistry. 2008;27(4):284–90.

[22] DeHaven CD, Evans AM, Dai H, Lawton KA. Organization of GC/MS and LC/MS metabolomics data into chemical libraries. Journal of Cheminformatics. 2010;2(1):9.

[23] Eppe G, Focant J-F, Pirard C, De Pauw E. PTV-LV-GC/MS/MS as screening and complementary method to HRMS for the monitoring of dioxin levels in food and feed. Talanta. 2004;63(5):1135–46.

[24] Canuto GA, da Cruz PL, Faccio AT, Klassen A, Tavares MF. Neglected diseases prioritized in Brazil under the perspective of metabolomics: a review. Electrophoresis. 2015;36(18):2336–47.

[25] Holmes E. The evolution of metabolic profiling in parasitology. Parasitology. 2010;137(09):1437–49.

[26] Furlong S. Unique roles for lipids in *Schistosoma mansoni*. Parasitology Today. 1991;7(2): 59–62.

[27] Ferreira MS, de Oliveira DN, de Oliveira RN, Allegretti SM, Catharino RR. Screening the life cycle of *Schistosoma mansoni* using high-resolution mass spectrometry. Analytica Chimica Acta. 2014;845:62–9.

[28] Retra K, Schmitz M, Yazdanbakhsh M, Tielens AG, Brouwers JF, van Hellemond JJ. The tegumental surface membranes of *Schistosoma mansoni* are enriched in parasite-specific phospholipid species. International Journal for Parasitology. 2015;45(9):629–36.

[29] Haslam SM, Morris HR, Dell A. Mass spectrometric strategies: providing structural clues for helminth glycoproteins. Trends in Parasitology. 2001;17(5):231–5.

[30] Smit CH, van Diepen A, Nguyen DL, Wuhrer M, Hoffmann KF, Deelder AM, et al. Glycomic analysis of life stages of the human parasite *Schistosoma mansoni* reveals developmental expression profiles of functional and antigenic glycan motifs. Molecular & Cellular Proteomics. 2015;14(7):1750–69.

[31] Khoo K-H, Chatterjee D, Caulfield JP, Morris HR, Dell A. Structural mapping of the glycans from the egg glycoproteins of *Schistosoma mansoni* and *Schistosoma japonicum*: identification of novel core structures and terminal sequences. Glycobiology. 1997;7(5): 663–77.

[32] Yoshioka L, Zanotti-Magalhães EM, Magalhães LA, Linhares AX. *Schistosoma mansoni*: estudo da patogenia da linhagem Santa Rosa (Campinas, SP, Brasil) em camundongos. Revista da Sociedade Brasileira de Medicina Tropical. 2002;35(3):203–7.

[33] Jang-Lee J, Curwen RS, Ashton PD, Tissot B, Mathieson W, Panico M, et al. Glycomics analysis of *Schistosoma mansoni* egg and cercarial secretions. Molecular & Cellular Proteomics. 2007;6(9):1485–99.

[34] Ferreira MS, Oliveira DN, Oliveira RN, Allegretti SM, Vercesi AE, Catharino RR. Mass spectrometry imaging: a new vision in differentiating *Schistosoma mansoni* strains. Journal of Mass Spectrometry. 2014;49(1):86–92.

[35] Meyer S, Van Liempt E, Imberty A, Van Kooyk Y, Geyer H, Geyer R, et al. DC-SIGN mediates binding of dendritic cells to authentic pseudo-LewisY glycolipids of *Schistosoma mansoni* cercariae, the first parasite-specific ligand of DC-SIGN. Journal of Biological Chemistry. 2005;280(45):37349–59.

[36] Wuhrer M, Dennis RD, Doenhoff MJ, Lochnit G, Geyer R. *Schistosoma mansoni* cercarial glycolipids are dominated by Lewis X and pseudo-Lewis Y structures. Glycobiology. 2000;10(1):89–101.

[37] Van Hellemond JJ, Retra K, Brouwers JF, van Balkom BW, Yazdanbakhsh M, Shoemaker CB, et al. Functions of the tegument of schistosomes: clues from the proteome and lipidome. International Journal for Parasitology. 2006;36(6):691–9.

[38] Pullan RL, Smith JL, Jasrasaria R, Brooker SJ. Global numbers of infection and disease burden of soil transmitted helminth infections in 2010. Parasites & Vectors. 2014;7(1):1.

[39] Malaria GH-DoPDa. The Burden of Ascariasis 2011 Available from: http://www.cdc.gov/globalhealth/ntd/diseases/ascaris_burden.html

[40] Committee WE. Prevention and Control of Schistosomiasis and Soil-Transmitted Helminthiasis. World Health Organization, Technical Report Series, No. 912; Geneva, Switzerland. 2002; vol. i–vi:1–57.

[41] Lo NC, Andrews JR, Bogoch II. Improving helminth treatment access: costs and opportunities. The Lancet Infectious Diseases. 2016;16(7):762–4.

[42] Organization WH. Investing to Overcome the Global Impact of Neglected Tropical Diseases: Third WHO Report on Neglected Diseases 2015. World Health Organization; Geneva, Switzerland. 2015.

[43] Shalaby HA. Anthelmintics resistance; how to overcome it? Iranian Journal of Parasitology. 2013;8(1):18.

[44] Albonico M, Engels D, Savioli L. Monitoring drug efficacy and early detection of drug resistance in human soil-transmitted nematodes: a pressing public health agenda for helminth control. International Journal for Parasitology. 2004;34(11):1205–10.

[45] Osei-Atweneboana MY, Eng JK, Boakye DA, Gyapong JO, Prichard RK. Prevalence and intensity of *Onchocerca volvulus* infection and efficacy of ivermectin in endemic communities in Ghana: a two-phase epidemiological study. The Lancet. 2007;369(9578):2021–9.

[46] Araujo P. Observations on the early ecdyses of larvae of *Ascaris lumbricoides, A. suum* and *Toxocara canis*. Revista do Instituto de Medicina Tropical de São Paulo. 1972;14(2):83–90.

[47] Artigas PdT, Ueta MT. About the evolution of *Ascaris lumbricoides* Linnaeus, 1758, in the larval stage inside the egg. Memories of Butantan Institute. 1989;51(1):15–24.

[48] Ligocka A, Paluszak Z. Effectiveness of different sanitization technologies on the inactivation of *Ascaris suum* eggs in organic waste. Bulletin of the Veterinary Institute in Pulawy. 2009;53:641–4.

[49] Ferreira MS, de Oliveira RN, de Oliveira DN, Esteves CZ, Allegretti SM, Catharino RR. Revealing praziquantel molecular targets using mass spectrometry imaging: an expeditious approach applied to *Schistosoma mansoni*. International Journal for Parasitology. 2015;45(6):385–91.

[50] Keiser J, Duthaler U, Utzinger J. Update on the diagnosis and treatment of food-borne trematode infections. Current Opinion in Infectious Diseases. 2010;23(5):513–20.

[51] Lima EdO, de Macedo CS, Esteves CZ, de Oliveira DN, Pessolani MCV, Nery JAdC, et al. Skin imprinting in silica plates: a potential diagnostic methodology for leprosy using high-resolution mass spectrometry. Analytical Chemistry. 2015;87(7):3585–92.

[52] Melo CFOR, Esteves CZ, de Oliveira RN, Guerreiro TM, de Oliveira DN, de Oliveira Lima E, et al. Early developmental stages of *Ascaris lumbricoides*. Parasitology Research. 2016. DOI: 10.1007/s00436-016-5183-2; 1–8.

[53] Dhanasekaran DN, Reddy EP. JNK signaling in apoptosis. Oncogene. 2008;27(48): 6245–51.

[54] Kumar A, Byun H-S, Bittman R, Saba JD. The sphingolipid degradation product trans-2-hexadecenal induces cytoskeletal reorganization and apoptosis in a JNK-dependent manner. Cellular Signalling. 2011;23(7):1144–52.

[55] Lin A, Dibling B. The true face of JNK activation in apoptosis. Aging Cell. 2002;1(2): 112–6.

[56] Golden JW, Riddle DL. A pheromone influences larval development in the nematode *Caenorhabditis elegans*. Science. 1982;218(4572):578–80.

[57] Dold C, Holland CV. Ascaris and ascariasis. Microbes and Infection. 2011;13(7):632–7.

[58] Hadley NF. Surface waxes and integumentary permeability: lipids deposited on or associated with the surface of terrestrial plants and animals help protect them from a lethal rate of desiccation. American Scientist. 1980;68(5):546–53.

[59] Niwa R, Niwa YS. Enzymes for ecdysteroid biosynthesis: their biological functions in insects and beyond. Bioscience, Biotechnology, and Biochemistry. 2014;78(8):1283–92.

[60] Qu Z, Kenny NJ, Lam HM, Chan TF, Chu KH, Bendena WG, et al. How did arthropod sesquiterpenoids and ecdysteroids arise? Comparison of hormonal pathway genes in noninsect arthropod genomes. Genome Biology and Evolution. 2015;7(7):1951–9.

[61] Entchev EV, Kurzchalia TV. Requirement of sterols in the life cycle of the nematode *Caenorhabditis elegans*. Seminars in Cell & Developmental Biology. 2005;16(2):175–182.

[62] Matyash V, Entchev EV, Mende F, Wilsch-Bräuninger M, Thiele C, Schmidt AW, et al. Sterol-derived hormone (s) controls entry into diapause in *Caenorhabditis elegans* by consecutive activation of DAF-12 and DAF-16. PLoS Biology. 2004;2(10):e280.

[63] Schlame M, Rua D, Greenberg ML. The biosynthesis and functional role of cardiolipin. Progress in Lipid Research. 2000;39(3):257–88.

[64] Takamiya S, Kita K, Wang H, Weinstein PP, Hiraishi A, Oya H, et al. Developmental changes in the respiratory chain of *Ascaris mitochondria*. Biochimica et Biophysica Acta (BBA)-Bioenergetics. 1993;1141(1):65–74.

[65] Guan XL, Cestra G, Shui G, Kuhrs A, Schittenhelm RB, Hafen E, et al. Biochemical membrane lipidomics during Drosophila development. Developmental Cell. 2013;24(1):98–111.

[66] Carlson D, Langley P, Huyton P. Sex Pheromone of the Tsetse Fly: Isolation, Identification, and Synthesis of Contact Aphrodisiacs. American Association for the Advancement of Science. Washington DC - USA. 1978.

[67] Steiger S, Schmitt T, Schaefer HM. The origin and dynamic evolution of chemical information transfer. Proceedings of the Royal Society of London B: Biological Sciences. 2010:rspb20102285.

[68] Brooker S, Kabatereine NB, Smith JL, Mupfasoni D, Mwanje MT, Ndayishimiye O, et al. An updated atlas of human helminth infections: the example of East Africa. International Journal of Health Geographics. 2009;8(1):1.

[69] Hotez PJ, Brindley PJ, Bethony JM, King CH, Pearce EJ, Jacobson J. Helminth infections: the great neglected tropical diseases. The Journal of Clinical Investigation. 2008;118(4): 1311–21.

[70] Rana AK, Misra-Bhattacharya S. Current drug targets for helminthic diseases. Parasitology Research. 2013;112(5):1819–31.

[71] Pink R, Hudson A, Mouriès M-A, Bendig M. Opportunities and challenges in antiparasitic drug discovery. Nature Reviews Drug Discovery. 2005;4(9):727–40.

[72] Renslo AR, McKerrow JH. Drug discovery and development for neglected parasitic diseases. Nature Chemical Biology. 2006;2(12):701–10.

[73] Geerts S, Gryseels B. Drug resistance in human helminths: current situation and lessons from livestock. Clinical Microbiology Reviews. 2000;13(2):207–22.

[74] van den Enden E. Pharmacotherapy of helminth infection. Expert Opinion on Pharmacotherapy. 2009;10(3):435–51.

[75] Hagel I, Giusti T. *Ascaris lumbricoides*: an overview of therapeutic targets. Infectious Disorders-Drug Targets (Formerly Current Drug Targets-Infectious Disorders). 2010;10(5):349–67.

[76] Hagel I, Cabrera M, Hurtado M, Sanchez P, Puccio F, Di Prisco M, et al. Infection by *Ascaris lumbricoides* and bronchial hyper reactivity: an outstanding association in Venezuelan school children from endemic areas. Acta Tropica. 2007;103(3):231–41.

[77] Stephenson LS, Latham MC, Ottesen E. Malnutrition and parasitic helminth infections. Parasitology. 2000;121(S1):S23–S38.

[78] Lacey E. The role of the cytoskeletal protein, tubulin, in the mode of action and mechanism of drug resistance to benzimidazoles. International Journal for Parasitology. 1988;18(7):885–936.

[79] Lacey E. Mode of action of benzimidazoles. Parasitology Today. 1990;6(4):112–5.

[80] Friedman PA, Platzer EG. Interaction of anthelmintic benzimidazoles and benzimidazole derivatives with bovine brain tubulin. Biochimica et Biophysica Acta (BBA)-General Subjects. 1978;544(3):605–14.

[81] Keiser J, Utzinger J. Efficacy of current drugs against soil-transmitted helminth infections: systematic review and meta-analysis. Jama. 2008;299(16):1937–48.

[82] Colley DG, Bustinduy AL, Secor WE, King CH. Human schistosomiasis. The Lancet. 2014;383(9936):2253–64.

[83] Steinmann P, Keiser J, Bos R, Tanner M, Utzinger J. Schistosomiasis and water resources development: systematic review, meta-analysis, and estimates of people at risk. The Lancet Infectious Diseases. 2006;6(7):411–25.

[84] Bygott J, Chiodini P. Praziquantel: neglected drug? Ineffective treatment? Or therapeutic choice in cystic hydatid disease? Acta Tropica. 2009;111(2):95–101.

[85] Gryseels B, Stelma F, Talla I, Van Dam G, Polman K, Sow S, et al. Epidemiology, immunology and chemotherapy of Schistosoma mansoni infections in a recently exposed community in Senegal. Tropical and Geographical Medicine. 1993;46(4 Spec No):209–19.

[86] De Vlas S, Gryseels B. Underestimation of *Schistosoma mansoni* prevalences. Parasitology Today. 1992;8(8):274–7.

[87] Gryseels B, de Vlas SJ. Worm burdens in schistosome infections. Parasitology Today. 1996;12(3):115–9.

[88] Doenhoff MJ. Is schistosomicidal chemotherapy sub-curative? Implications for drug resistance. Parasitology Today. 1998;14(10):434–5.

[89] Peng J, Yang Y, Feng X, Cheng G, Lin J. Molecular characterizations of an inhibitor of apoptosis from *Schistosoma japonicum*. Parasitology Research. 2010;106(4):967–76.

[90] Meier H, Blaschke G. Investigation of praziquantel metabolism in isolated rat hepatocytes. Journal of Pharmaceutical and Biomedical Analysis. 2001;26(3):409–15.

[91] van Balkom BW, van Gestel RA, Brouwers JF, Krijgsveld J, Tielens AG, Heck AJ, et al. Mass spectrometric analysis of the *Schistosoma mansoni* tegumental sub-proteome. Journal of Proteome Research. 2005;4(3):958–66.

[92] Pinto-Almeida A, Mendes T, de Oliveira RN, Corrêa SdAP, Allegretti SM, Belo S, et al. Morphological characteristics of *Schistosoma mansoni* PZQ-resistant and-susceptible strains are different in presence of Praziquantel. Frontiers in Microbiology. 2016;7:11.

Chapter 3

Helminths and their Role in Environmental Engineering

Blanca Jiménez, Catalina Maya, José A. Barrios and
Inés Navarro

Additional information is available at the end of the chapter

http://dx.doi.org/10.5772/64878

Abstract

Helminth eggs represent an important challenge to environmental engineers as they are among the most difficult biological parasites to inactivate in wastewater and sludge. Even though no official data on helminthiasis exist, it is estimated that more than 2.6 billion people are affected. These parasites are of concern in developing countries, particularly in those areas where the reuse of wastewater and sludge for agriculture is common. With regard to this, the unrestricted use of wastewater for irrigation presents a serious health risk due to the dissemination of pathogens, particularly helminth eggs. Helminth eggs survive in water, soil, and crops for several months and over much longer periods than other microorganisms. Therefore, and in order to minimize risk, several guidelines and regulations exist which limit their content in wastewater and sludge. Risk assessment estimates that such regulations may be less strict in developing countries where higher concentrations of helminth eggs occur in wastewater and sludge. These eggs need to be removed from wastewater and inactivated in sludge using certain treatment processes, some of which are not feasible in developing countries. Adequate methods are needed to precisely identify and quantify helminth eggs in environmental samples. Therefore, a multidisciplinary approach is needed to address helminthiasis in environmental engineering issues.

Keywords: Biosolids, guidelines and regulations, helminth eggs, helminthiasis, inactivation processes, microbial risk assessment, wastewater

1. Introduction

For centuries, wastewater has been used for agricultural irrigation throughout the world, and this is still a common practice in several countries. There are many examples that show wastewater reuse is key to increasing food production and improving local economies. This is simply due to the high water demand for irrigation. In developing countries, this amounts to 81% of the total water extracted and to around 45% in developed countries [1]. As an example, in Mexico, where 75% of the territory is semiarid, wastewater reuse for agriculture is often practiced. Mexican farmers have long appreciated wastewater use because it contains, in addition to water, organic matter, nitrogen, and phosphorus, which act as fertilizers, increasing crop yield. Jiménez [2] summarized the reasons why wastewater is reused for irrigation: (a) it significantly saves fresh water; (b) it provides nutrients to soil; (c) it reduces or eliminates the need for chemical fertilizers; (d) it contributes to the expansion of agricultural land in arid and semi-arid areas; (e) it increases farmers' income; and (f) it is a relatively cheap disposal method for wastewater, reducing surface water pollution. It is estimated that there are 20 million hectares in at least 50 developing countries where wastewater is used to irrigate [3], representing around 10% of the total irrigated land. Even though the reuse of wastewater for agricultural irrigation has several benefits, it poses a public health risk due its pathogenic content. Among these pathogens, helminth eggs are of particular concern.

Helminths are parasitic worms transmitted to humans via their eggs (infective life stage, **Figure 1**). They are considered to be the biological structures most resistant to inactivation in the environmental engineering field [4]. Most helminths are transmitted by direct contact with contaminated soil, crops, or wastewater (e.g., *Ascaris lumbricoides*, *Trichuris trichiura*, and hookworms), but some require the presence of intermediate hosts (e.g., freshwater snails in the case of schistosomiasis) [5].

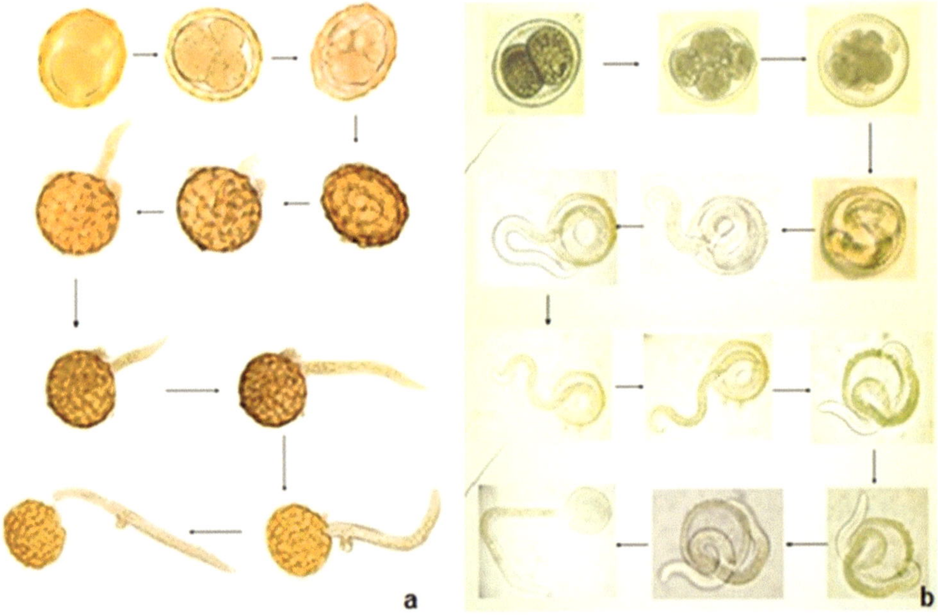

Figure 1. Fertilized eggs with larval growth and development of the worm for (a) *Ascaris lumbricoides* and (b) *Toxocara canis* (Photographic archives, Treatment and Reuse Group, Instituto de Ingeniería, UNAM).

Concerns about their presence are related to their very low infectious dose, their high rate of survival in the environment for extended periods of time (up to several years, compared to weeks for other pathogens), and their high resistance to conventional disinfection processes [6]. Helminth eggs are a particular threat to health where sanitation conditions are poor, polluted water is used for irrigation, or where excreta or non-treated sludge is disposed of in an uncontrolled manner. They cause a set of diseases call "helminthiasis" that are given specific names based on the genera involved (for instance, ascariasis for genus *Ascaris*). Symptoms include deterioration of the intestines, toxic effects, blood loss, diarrhea, undernourishment, and anemia. Some helminths gnaw away at the intestinal wall causing hemorrhages while simultaneously secreting an anti-coagulant. The damage caused by inflammation, and the wounds they open generate tumors and excrescences. In addition, helminths can block conduits (for example, biliary) or cause intestinal obstruction and perforation of the digestive tract causing peritonitis [6, 7].

Helminthiases may lead to serious collateral effects limiting the physical and mental development of children, notably when repeated infection occurs between 5 and 15 years of age. It is estimated that 182 million children of preschool age are infected, that is, around 33% of those living in developing countries [8–10]. These children display lower height and weight due to undernourishment compared to well-nourished children living in healthy environments. At the same time, malnutrition results in a low school performance and a decrease in intelligence quotient (IQ) [11, 12]. Other effects, such as epileptic seizures, violent headaches, vertigo, local paralysis, vomiting, and optical and physical perturbations have been reported [7].

In spite of that, the control of helminth eggs was neglected until the late 1980s when the World Health Organization (WHO) developed guidelines for water and sludge reuse in agriculture. In 2006 the World Health Organization [6] confirmed the need to control the associated health hazards through an updated version of the guidelines for safe use of wastewater, excreta, and sludge in agriculture and aquaculture. These guidelines recommend limiting the helminth egg content in wastewater, excreta, and sludge; however, to achieve this, it is necessary to remove and inactivate the eggs. The following sections discuss the data collected for helminth eggs in environmental matrices, public health risks, regulations in different countries, treatment methods for wastewater and sludge, and analytical methods to determine their concentrations in environmental matrices.

2. Helminth egg content in wastewater and sludge

Helminths are multi-cellular organisms (worms) with a wide variety of shapes and sizes. Some of them are free-living (like earthworms), while others are parasites. Helminths can be classified in different ways, but the classification most frequently used considers their body shape. Roundworms are called Nematodes while flatworms are called Plathelminthes; if the latter have segments then are referred to as Cestodes while non-segmented ones are termed Trematodes [5]. As mentioned previously, helminths reproduce via the production of eggs, which are microscopic structures whose shape, size (20–180 m), and density (1.06–1.23) vary.

A fertilized *Ascaris lumbricoides* female roundworm can lay around 200,000 eggs per day and up to 27,000,000 eggs over a lifespan of 10–24 months, while the *Taenia saginata*, a beef tapeworm, can produce as many as 800,000 eggs per segment per day (a typically sized worm may have around 1000 segments) [13–15]. Helminth eggs contained in wastewater, sludge, or excreta may be viable (alive) but not infective. To be infective, the eggs need to develop into larvae, which require a temperature of around 25°C combined with a moisture content of at least 5% [16]. These conditions are found in soils or crops where eggs develop into larvae within a few days, remaining viable for several months or years [6]. In addition, infective doses are very low, within the range of 1–10 eggs. Most helminthiases are, therefore, transmitted via the eggs through a human-water-soil-crop-human pathway.

The content of helminth eggs in developing countries' wastewater and sludge differs considerably from that of developed ones (**Table 1**). Helminth egg concentrations may be 7–80 times greater in developing countries. For instance, the helminth egg content in developing countries ranges from 70 to 3000 helminth eggs per liter (HE/L) in wastewater and 70–735 helminth eggs per gram of total dry solids (HE/g TS) in sludge. In comparison, for developed countries, the content in wastewater is only 1–9 HE/L and that for sludge is 2–13 HE/g TS [17]. Not all eggs are viable, but, in general, mean viability generally reaches 88%, with an even higher percentage for *Ascaris* spp. (90%) as a result of their high environmental resistance [4, 18, 19].

Country/region	Helminth eggs in wastewater (HE/L)	Helminth eggs in sludge (HE/g TS)	References
Developing countries	70–3000	67–735	[13, 18, 20]
Tropical countries		300–3000	[18]
Brazil	166–202	1–76	[21]
Cayman islands	100–1230		[14]
China	840	2300	[22]
France	9	5–7	[20]
Egypt (liquid primary)	6–42	Mean: 67, Max: 735	[23–24]
Egypt (dewatered primary)		Mean: 8, Max: 124	[24]
Ghana		76	[20, 24]
Germany		<1	
Great Britain		<6	
Japan	80	1–51	[25]
Jordan	300		[14]
Mexico	6–98 (up to 330 in poor areas)	73–177 (viable eggs)	[17]
Morocco	840		[26]
South Africa	772	2–40	[27, 28]
Syria	800		[29]
Tunisia	30		[15]
Ukraine	60		[13]
United States of America	1–8	2–13	[20]

Table 1. Helminth ova content in wastewater and sludge for selected countries.

3. Prevalence of helminthiasis

Stoll N. [30] calculated that there were 2200 million nematode infections worldwide and predicted that by 1991, there would be 5000 million infected people. Similarly, he estimated that the Chinese population produced a total of 18,000 tons of *Ascaris* eggs per year. Currently, it is estimated that more than 2.6 billion people are infected with helminths (**Table 2**), and although helminthiases are globally distributed, the prevalence of disease is mostly limited to developing countries [5, 7, 31]. They are endemic in regions of Africa, Central America, South America, and the Far East, with incidence rates as high as 90% for specific regions and sectors of the population [6, 7]. The dominant species depends on local conditions. However, most of the information related to procedures to control helminth eggs in sludge was gathered in developed countries where the low concentrations found render it difficult to utilize the data collected [20].

Around 96% of the helminthiases reported are induced by infection by Nematoda and Trematoda classes, with 4% due to Cestoda [5, 32]. The most common genus is *Ascaris lumbricoides* [33] with more than 819 million people infected. The eggs are highly infective (commonly, one egg suffices), very persistent in the environment, and very resistant to conventional disinfection/inactivation processes [10–12, 34]. For example, embryonated eggs of *Ascaris* spp. can survive for 20 days at temperatures of -20.9 to -27°C and survive in frozen Siberian soils for 10 years [35]. This resistance comes from the fact that eggs are surrounded by a series of layers functioning as a barrier that protects the larva against harsh environmental conditions. Indeed, the different helminth egg species possess 3–4 layers with different physical and chemical characteristics: (a) The 1–2 outer layers are formed of mucopolysaccharides and proteins; (b) the middle layers have chitin which provides structure and mechanical resistance; and (c) the inner layer, composed of lipids and proteins, protect the egg from desiccation, strong acid and bases, oxidants, reductive agents, detergents and proteolytic compounds [36–39].

The interaction of the layers' components with external agents may cause a change in their chemical composition, as well as in the specific function of each layer, which in turn modifies their permeability, their mechanical and chemical resistance and, finally, the egg viability. These mechanisms may be similar to those that take place during the hatching process, during which the larva secretes certain enzymes that induce the loss of permeability of the ascaroside layer and attack the outer eggshell layers. However, in this case, the layer remains intact until the hatching of the larva with no detectable chemical change [40–41].

The impact on the quality of life of infected populations may be illustrated using an estimation made in 2013 for years lived with disabiliy (YLDs) [42]. This amounted worldwide to 1,004,000 years for anemia caused by hookworm disease, and 671,000 years for schistosomiasis. Based on the analysis of YLDs estimates, ascariasis was among the eight most prevalent causes of disease, affecting more than 10% of world's population in 2013, such that if the mean prevalence of chronic sequelae is selected, for periods longer than 3 months, the impact of ascariasis was estimated in 819 million cases.

Helminth species	Common name	Prevalence (million inhabitants)	Regional presence
Nematoda			
Ascaris lumbricoides	Roundworm	819	Many regions of South-East Asia, Africa, and Central and South America
Ancylostoma duodenale	Hookworm	439	Tropical and subtropical countries (Sub-Saharan Africa), Central and South America, the Caribbean, Asia and in the Pacific islands
Necator americanus			
Strongyloides stercoralis		370	
Trichuris trichiura	Whipworm	465	Moist, warm, tropical regions of Asia, Africa, Central and South America, and the Caribbean islands
Trichostrongylus orientalis	Roundworm	Several	Mainly rural communities in Asia
Cestoda			
Hymenolepis diminuta	Rat tapeworm	50	Most occurrences in areas which lack adequate sanitation but may be found around the world in South America, Southeast Asia, Western Africa and East Africa; and in areas of the tropics and subtropics and some areas of Southern and Eastern Europe, the United States of America and Mexico.
Hymenolepis nana	Dwarf tapeworm		
Taenia saginata	Beef tapeworm	50	
Taenia solium	Pork tapeworm		
Trematoda			
Schistosoma mansoni	Blood fluke	207	Tropical and subtropical regions. This species occurs widely throughout Africa and South America, especially in Brazil, Venezuela, Surinam, Guyana and several Caribbean islands, including Puerto Rico, St. Lucia, Martinique, and Guadalupe
Clonorchis sinensis *Echinostoma* spp. *Fasciola gigantica* *Fasciola hepatica* *Fasciolopsis buski* *Heterophyes* spp. *Metagonimus* spp. *Opisthorchis felineus* *Opisthorchis viverrini* *Paragonimus* spp.	Food-borne Trematodes	56	Largely in Southern and Eastern Asia but also in Central and Eastern Europe.
Fasciolopsis buski	Intestinal fluke		
Other groups		100	Worldwide
Total		Over 2.6 billion infections worldwide	

Source: Ref. [5].

Table 2. Common helminth species and helminthiasis by region.

4. Guidelines and regulations

As mentioned previously, the use of domestic wastewater for irrigation, even without treatment, is an established practice in many countries. However, it leads to the proliferation of helminthiasis in the exposed population [6, 43]. Following a series of epidemiological studies, since 1989, the World Health Organization has recommended a limit for the content of nematode eggs in wastewater reused for agricultural irrigation [44]. Similarly, sludge produced during wastewater treatment may be reused in agriculture or soil remediation after adequate treatment to reduce its microbial content. Once treated, wastewater and sludge need

http://dx.doi.org/10.5772/64878

to meet national regulations or international criteria in order to be safely reused. For instance, in 2006, the World Health Organization suggested that a limit of less than 1 viable helminth egg per liter (HE/L) in wastewater makes it acceptable for agricultural reuse, while less than 1 viable helminth egg per gram of total dry solids (1 HE/g TS) is required in sludge [6]. However, these limits are difficult to meet in countries or regions with endemic diseases, requiring effective inactivation processes to control the high concentrations of helminth eggs.

Following the WHO guidelines [6], many countries have set standards for helminth eggs in treated water, including Brazil, Colombia, Costa Rica, Chile, Israel, Jordan, Mexico, Saudi Arabia, and Tunisia. These standards also set recommendations for the types of crops to be irrigated, irrigation methods, and other intervention measures to manage risks. In addition, sludge and biosolids (treated sludge) regulations have been developed by several countries, led principally by the United States (**Tables 3** and **4**).

Country	Regulation-standard-guidelines	Type	Helminth eggs limit, eggs/L
Australia	Australian regulations, 1995	U	–
		N/A	Absent
Argentina	Resolución 778/96	U	–
		R	<1 Nematode
Chile	Norma 1333 (1978)	U	-
		R	<1 Nematode
Mexico	NOM-001-SEMARNAT-1996	U	<1
		R	<5
United States of America	Department of Health Services (DHS), California, 1918.	N/A	Absent
WHO	WHO, 2006	U	≤1 (arithmetic mean)
		R	
		Localized (drip) irrigation)	Low-growing crops: ≤1 (arithmetic mean) High-growing crops: no recommendation

U: Unrestricted irrigation: For agricultural irrigation of all kinds of crops, including those that are eaten uncooked (lettuce, onion); R: Restricted irrigation: For agricultural irrigation of all kinds of crops, except that are eaten uncooked (highly mechanized, labor intensive).

[a]When children under 15 years of age are exposed, additional health protection measures should be used (e.g., treatment to ≤0.1 egg per liter, protective equipment such as gloves or shoes /boots or chemical treatment);

[b]An arithmetic mean should be determined throughout the irrigation season. The mean value of ≤1 egg per liter should be obtained for at least 90% of samples in order to allow for the occasional high-value sample (i.e., with >10 eggs per liter). In some wastewater treatment processes (e.g., waste stabilization ponds), the hydraulic retention time can be used as a surrogate to assure compliance with a limit of ≤ 1 egg per liter;

[c]Including fruit trees and olives, not crops harvested directly from the soil.
Source: Refs. [6, 45–47].

Table 3. Regulations for helminth egg content in treated wastewater use in agriculture.

Country	Regulation standard guidelines	Class/type	Helminth egg limit, eggs/g TS
Brazil	CONAMA 375/2006	A	0.25
		B	10
Chile	No. 123 (30/08/2006)	A	0.25
		B	-
France	Directive 86/278	-	0.3
Mexico	NOM-004-SEMARNAT-2002	A	1
		B	10
		C	35
New Zealand	Guidelines for the safe application of biosolids to land in New Zealand	A	0.25
Norway	Regulations for the treatment, use and disposal of sewage sludge	–	Absent
South Africa	Guidelines for the utilisation and disposal of wastewater sludge (Vol. 2)	A	0.25
		B	1
The United States of America	CFR 40 Part 503 /1993	A	0.25
The WHO	WHO, 2006		1

[V]Viable eggs.

Table 4. Regulations for helminth egg content in sludge.

In general, the standard values have been set to protect human health, allowing sludge application at sites where human contact may occur [48]. Under those conditions, a value of <1 HE/g is to be achieved (Class A). Only Brazil and Mexico allow higher concentrations of helminth eggs. However, in the case of Brazil, the regulation states that Class B sludge may be land applied only after risk assessment determines that this is a secure practice. In contrast, the limits for Class B and C sludge in the Mexican regulations refer to total eggs, assuming not all of them are viable, and is intended for land application without human contact (e.g., agriculture, soil restoration, forestry). However, to enforce these limits, it is necessary to correctly measure the helminth egg content in wastewater and sludge (treated or untreated).

5. Quantitative microbial risk assessment (QMRA)

WHO guidelines and US EPA limits for helminth eggs were based on limited epidemiological evidences, and on the performance of different sludge treatment methods, rather than the results of a risk assessment. Neither of the organizations based their considerations on results of a dose response-curve "because methodologies had not been developed sufficiently enough to make such calculations" [6, 49]. As a result, no human risk assessment was conducted, due to the lack of a dose-response model appropriate to describe helminth eggs infection. At the time, of the three different methods used to evaluate microbial risks: microbiology laboratory analysis, epidemiological studies, and quantitative microbial risk assessment (QMRA), only the first two have been applied to helminth data [50–52]. In contrast, a number of human dose-response relationships have been developed for bacteria, viruses, and protozoa [53–59]; consequently, a dose-response function for helminth infections was required for applying a QMRA.

QMRA is a modeling approach used to predict the human health risks from exposure to pathogens and has been shown to be effective in assessing the transmission of water and food-borne infections. It estimates the risk of infection or illness based on the concentration of infectious pathogens in wastewater, on surfaces or in drinking water, or from other environmental sources (e.g., crops, biosolids, air), the estimated ingestion rate, and the established dose-response models for a given population.

Since 2009 a dose-response curve is only available for *Ascaris* [60], although other helminths genus are highly relevant in wastewater and sludge reuse, especially in developing countries [61]. This curve was derived from *A. lumbricoides* prevalence data obtained from stools of a large sample of children in the Mezquital Valley in Mexico, rather than conducting human *Ascaris* dose-challenge studies. Navarro et al. [60] found that their *Ascaris* infection data best fitted the β-Poisson dose-response equation [Eq. (1)].

$$P(d)=1-\left[1+\left(d/N_{50}\right)\left(2^{1/\alpha}-1\right)\right]^{-\alpha} \quad (1)$$

where P(d) is the risk of infection in an individual who has ingested *d Ascaris* eggs on one occasion; N_{50} is the mean *Ascaris* infective dose; and α is an *Ascaris* 'infectivity constant'. They found the values of N_{50} and α to be 859 and 0.104, respectively.

Use of the QMRA tool allowed an initial target estimation of *Ascaris* concentration in sludge and wastewater. These values were greater than WHO and US EPA limits [62], but with an estimated probability of infection smaller than the prevalence rate observed on site. Such scenarios may allow a gradual improvement in population health conditions, as well as working towards an *Ascaris* eggs content in sludge and/or wastewater which gradually should approach regulation limits. The authors concluded from these risk analyses that regulations targeting biosolids reuse in developing countries should address the challenge of firstly deciding an acceptable infection risk and, secondly, putting in place an integrated framework for risk management, involving additional health protection measures. They suggested factors to be considered, which include, amongst others: (a) an affordable treatment process, (b) crop restriction policy, (c) different sludge application rates, and (d) efficient produce washing methods.

Further research should focus on QMRAs with the β-Poisson dose-response model for *Ascaris lumbricoides*, which have demonstrated through case studies its application to analyze the tolerable risk and to evaluate additional control measures, considered as potential interventions for health risk reduction. They illustrates the importance of two recommendations from WHO guidelines [3]: The first is that in some circumstances, "it is recommended that, initially, a national standard is established for a locally appropriate level of tolerable additional burden of disease based on the local incidence of diarrheal disease," and the second that post-treatment health-protection control measures can achieve significant pathogen reductions, so that wastewater treatment does not have to achieve the total pathogen reduction required to protect consumer health.

In the first case, it was shown that a maximum tolerable additional disability-adjusted life year (DALY) loss per person per year (pppy) of 10^{-4} is an appropriate value, especially in low-income countries [63]. It is more applicable than the WHO guidelines [3] default value of $\leq 10^{-6}$ DALY loss for the tolerable additional burden of disease due to wastewater pathogens. A tolerable *Ascaris* infection risk of 1.2×10^{-2} [64] corresponds to a tolerable DALY loss of 10^{-4} pppy. Therefore, the QMRA results, applying the β-Poisson dose-response model, indicate that a ova reduction to 10 eggs/L results in a risk of $\sim 3 \times 10^{-3}$, which could be used as a guideline value. This is in agreement with previous recommendations of ≤15 eggs/L [65, 66] who also suggested that pathogen reduction may be achieved by simple wastewater treatment.

QMRA applications using the β-Poisson dose-response model have illustrated the health protection levels that may be achieved with some control measures. Experimental work by [67] showed that a waiting period of 120 days at 25°C or 90 days at 37°C following land application of biosolids to lettuce fields would result in acceptable yearly risks of less than 10^{-4} for *Ascaris* for the planting of the crop and acceptable yearly risks of less than 10^{-4} for *Ascaris* from the consumption of lettuce. They were able to evaluate the effect of different incubation temperatures of biosolids on the inactivation of *Ascaris* eggs and estimated an appropriate time between the application of biosolids to land and the harvesting of lettuce to achieve an acceptable risk for consumers at the end of the exposure pathway.

An important topic with regard to the safe use of wastewater in agriculture is the estimation of the number of days of irrigation cessation required to achieve tolerable annual infection risk. The on-site die-off of pathogens through irrigation cessation is considered a potential intervention for health risk reduction. Seidu et al. [68] undertook the challenge of comparing the best fit die-off model for *Ascaris* derived in their study with existing die-off models in a QMRA. The β-Poisson dose-response model was used in order to assess the effect of different die-off models on the days required to achieve the tolerable annual infection risk associated with the consumption of wastewater-irrigated lettuce. The study showed that none of the survival curves of *Ascaris suum* fitted the log-linear model, indicating that the classical first-order kinetic approach is inadequate in many cases. The implication of using die-off models for health risk assessment was an underestimation of the number of days of irrigation cessation necessary to reduce *Ascaris* infection risk for the log-linear die-off rate compared to the biphasic die-off rate of their study. Therefore, cessation of irrigation as a health risk reduction measure appeared to be impractical, given the prevailing conditions, in their study area. This also indicated that assessing the health risk reduction efficacy of intervention using QMRA models is dependent on accurate characterization of the die-off of pathogenic organisms.

Studies of Barker *et al* [69] and Kundu *et al* [70] assessed the risk of gastrointestinal infections caused by *Ascaris lumbricoides*, among other pathogens, associated with the consumption of raw vegetables. They used a QMRA in two developing regions (Kumasi, Ghana, and the Arias-Arenales River, Argentina). Both studies are examples of risk estimations that consider the *Ascaris* infection risk as a result of the quality of the water resource used for irrigation, the results after harvesting, and due to crops being eaten raw. They also included the *Ascaris* infection risk from accidental ingestion of contaminated water and produce washing behaviors of the population. They developed different approaches for following the steps of a QMRA, showing that a wide range of assumptions may be made for specific exposure scenarios to identify the reduction measures needed to protect human health. Their results and discussion also made it evident that the variability observed is a consequence of the inherent characteristics of each case study and that the uncertainties analyzed in the different scenarios illustrated the variables that played a major role in the risk estimates. Barker et al. [69] concluded that "particularly in the context of developing countries, it is important to balance the risks with the benefits of access to fresh vegetables. It is important that the consideration of the benefits is not lost in the discussion of the risks, which remain real and significant".

Finally, it was shown that these case studies illustrate that QMRA is a useful tool for developing standards for human exposure to pathogens. Clearly, additional interventions and changes in behavior need to be investigated and implemented to reduce the risks to acceptable levels; however, in the meantime, a more efficient and rapid analytical technique of helminth egg detection in environmental samples is needed, as well as high-quality control of local data to improve the exposure scenarios.

6. Wastewater treatment processes

In order to remove helminth eggs from wastewater, processes that remove particles, such as sedimentation, filtration, or coagulation-flocculation, are employed [71–73]. In practice, and in contrast to other microorganisms, helminth ova cannot be inactivated with chlorine, UV light, or ozone (in the latter case at least not with economical doses since a concentration of >36 mg/L ozone is required with 1 h of contact time). As discussed previously, their morphology, in terms of their external structure, protects them from inactivation.

The main removal mechanisms employed during wastewater treatment are associated with the size and density of helminth eggs. Since they are denser than water, they may be correlated with solid particles in wastewater [measured as total suspended solids (TSS)] and this, therefore, aids their separation. This correlation is used to indirectly measure their content and evaluate the performance of treatment processes in terms of their removal [74]. Due to their size and adhesiveness, helminth eggs can also be removed from wastewater through filtration [33, 71, 75, 76]. In terms of wastewater treatment, the following processes may achieve good removal of helminth eggs [33, 73].

- *Stabilization ponds (SP).* Stabilization ponds are large shallow basins enclosed by earth embankments, in which raw wastewater is treated by entirely natural processes. Several factors contribute to removing helminths, namely sedimentation, temperature, sunlight, pH, microorganism predation, adsorption, and absorption, although sedimentation is the most effective. There are three types of SP: anaerobic, facultative, and maturation ponds. Anaerobic (1-day retention time) and facultative ponds (5–15 days) are best for helminth ova removal.

- *Reservoirs*. Similarly to stabilization ponds, reservoirs and dams can remove helminth ova from wastewater if retention times longer than 20 days are used.
- *Coagulation-flocculation*. This process promotes aggregation of solid particles with the use of metallic salts (mainly alum or iron salts) and produces water suitable for agricultural reuse. When this process uses low coagulant doses (50–65 mg/L) combined with synthetic polymers as flocculants (0.8–1.2 mg/L), it is called chemical enhanced primary treatment (CEPT) or advanced primary treatment (APT). CEPT or APT promote particle aggregation, including helminth eggs, into flocs that increase their settling velocity and allow separation via sedimentation.
- *Filtration*. This consists of passing primary or secondary effluent through a porous material that retains the solids and produces a good quality effluent. Rapid filtration (rate >2 m/h) is one of the most useful treatments to remove helminth eggs from effluents, either physicochemical or biological, with values consistently below 1 HE/L.
- *Constructed wetlands*. These are designed to operate by gravity, and they are generally shallow to allow a better removal of pollutants. The plants typically used are as follows: (a) large plants with floating or aerial leaves; (b) plants with well-developed and submerged roots, such as rushes, water hyacinth, reeds, and water lilies; and (c) very small floating plants with few roots or no roots at all, such as those of the *Lamenacea* family, *Lemna* or duckweed, *Spirodela, Wolffia, Wolffiela*, and *Salvinia* [77, 78]. Most of the removal of helminth eggs occurs within the first 25 m in a horizontal flow gravel bed wetland (100 m long), reaching 100% after the entire process [79, 80].

7. Sludge stabilization

Once separated from wastewater, most helminth eggs are concentrated in sludge, which needs to be adequately treated before its land application or disposal. Since helminth eggs are the most resistant form of the parasites [4, 18–19], sludge treatment processes must consider their initial concentrations to achieve their inactivation and comply with regulations. In this respect, helminth eggs have the ability to survive for long periods of time in raw sludge and soil (up to 6 years from their initial application [81]). As a result, different sludge treatment processes may be used to inactivate helminth eggs, often including thermal treatment.

As an example, some of the best results for helminth egg inactivation in sludge have been obtained using thermal treatment at 108°C, irradiation at 1000 Gy or greater, pasteurization at 70°C, and thermophilic (55°C) anaerobic digestion [82–85]. In addition, the US EPA [48] allows the use of different alternatives to produce a sludge that meets class A limits (<0.25 HE/g TS) which include processes such as composting, irradiation, pasteurization, and heat treatment. However, all these advanced treatments require investments that are not always feasible in developing countries, where basic sanitation strategies are of greater importance.

With respect to more conventional treatment processes, mesophilic aerobic or anaerobic digestion do not reduce viable eggs of *Ascaris, Trichuris, Toxocara,* or *Capillaria* [84]. When mesophilic anaerobic digestion has been evaluated, at least 50% of *Ascaris suum* eggs were found to survive for up to 5 weeks [86]. In contrast, studies of alkaline pre- and post-stabilization with 40% (w/w) lime [71, 87] have reported inactivation efficiencies between 92 and 95%.

Several studies have evaluated the combination of different adverse conditions to inactivate helminth eggs, with some of them including the use of a range of chemicals. For example, Ghiglietti *et al* [88] found that a combination of sludge alkalinization with ammonium hydroxide (NH_4OH) at 30°C causes the inactivation of *A. lumbricoides, A. suum,* and *Trichuris muris*, and that a temperature of 40°C, with or without ammonia, was unfavorable for the development of the eggs; however, at 22°C, there was no effect, even with the addition of ammonia. Another study [87] also obtained a 69% reduction of viable helminth eggs after 2 h contact time with 10% (w/w) ammonia. When 50% ammonia was added, inactivation reached 94%. In addition, optimal conditions for egg inactivation have been found to include a combination of temperature, pH, and dryness of the sludge (45°C, pH of 5.3 and 90% dryness within 6 days or 45°C, pH of 12.7 and 90% dryness within 19 days) [4]. These results also confirm that the acidification process with peracetic acid was more effective than lime treatment. In this respect, Barrios *et al* [89] also evaluated the use of peracetic acid for microbial inactivation in sludge; results showed that the application of 550 ppm for 30 min reduced viable helminth eggs by 94% from an initial concentration of 93 viable HE/g TS. Aguilar et al. [90] evaluated the use of silver for inactivating high concentrations of helminth eggs in sludge (168–215 viable HE/g TS); the use of silver alone was not sufficient for complete inactivation. However, when silver was applied with copper and a synergistic agent (5:50:13.3 mg Ag–Cu–SA/g TS), total inactivation was achieved after 60 min.

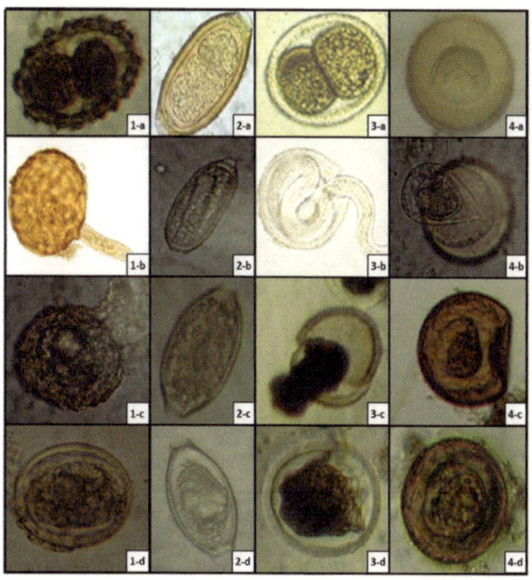

Figure 2. Viable eggs: 1-a *Ascaris;* 2-a *Trichuris;* 3-a, *Toxocara;* and 4-a *Hymenolepis diminuta*. Larval eggs: 1-b *Ascaris;* 2-b *Trichuris;* 3-b *Toxocara;* 4-b *Hymenolepis*. Morphological damage observed when eggs were subjected to different chemical reagents: 1-c and 1-d *Ascaris;* 2-c and 2-d *Trichuris;* 3-c and 3-d *Toxocara;* and 4-c and 4-d *Hymenolepis*. (Photographic archives, Treatment and Reuse Group, Instituto de Ingeniería, UNAM.).

Following some of those studies, the effect of different chemicals on the morphology of helminth eggs has been evaluated. After the addition of peracetic acid, lime, increased temperature, and desiccation, serious malformations of the embryos and larva, and even the destruction of the embryo, have been documented (**Figure 2**).

8. Analytical techniques

In order to quantify helminth eggs in wastewater, sludge, and excreta, an analytical procedure based on their visual identification and enumeration is used. However, current methodologies are not always effective for identification since experienced technicians are required, and therefore, results are often neither accurate nor reliable. Moreover, there is no universally accepted method to quantify them in sludge and biosolids [91]. The available analytical procedures commonly have two steps: (a) the separation of as many eggs as possible from other particles in the sample and (b) their visual identification under the microscope, where the concentrated sediment (pellet) contains many other types of particles. Only a properly trained technician is able to discriminate such particles from the eggs, and this technician has to visually identify the different species of helminth eggs. This is critical and constitutes the main source of error and uncertainty in the methodology. In particular, it is problematic when processing samples with a high content of helminth eggs because the discrimination process is tedious and time-consuming. In short, the challenge for the analysis is to separate, correctly identify, and enumerate helminth eggs in samples that, even after processing, contain many impurities, which render this difficult. Several alternative methods have been proposed to quantify helminths, considering the complexity of dealing with environmental samples. However, the efficacy of their application is yet to be proven.

As part of newly proposed analytical techniques, molecular methods have reported variable results. Some of these have been tested with synthetic samples and as a result, they still need to demonstrate their feasibility where actual environmental samples are analyzed. A recent study [92] compared different methods to detect hookworm ova over a range of concentrations and concluded that direct DNA extraction exhibited some limitations due to polymerase chain reaction (PCR) inhibitors present in environmental samples. In contrast, another study reported a sensitivity of one to four hookworm ova in wastewater samples [93]. Using quantitative PCR methods, *Ascaris* eggs may be detected [94, 95]; however, this technique still has some limitations, such as the low recovery rates obtained in samples with low numbers of eggs or the production of false positives.

A recent approach has proposed the use of image processing algorithms to identify and quantify helminth eggs from photographs taken using a microscope. This method is based on selected characteristics of helminth eggs that allow their correct identification without the need for a highly trained technician; it is capable of identifying up to eight species of helminths with a specificity (capacity to discriminate between species of helminth eggs and other objects) and sensitivity (capacity to correctly identify and classify the different species of helminth eggs) of 0.99 and 0.90, respectively [5].

9. Final remarks

Much knowledge has been gained since the early 80s but there are still major challenges in the field of environmental engineering. A large number of species of helminth eggs are excreted by humans and are discharged into wastewater, representing a significant source of pollution to the environment. In particular, when untreated or partially treated wastewater is discharged or used for agriculture, the risk of transmitting these types of diseases increases. The concentrations of helminth eggs in environmental matrices (wastewater and sludge) are directly related to public health. Therefore, until the millennium goals of 100% sanitation worldwide are met, about 2.6 billion cases of helminthiasis will prevail. Meanwhile the integrated management of wastewater and sludge remains as an engineering challenge.

Wastewater and sludge regulations focus on public health protection, assuming agricultural reuse and land application is practiced. Very low concentrations are permitted in treated effluents and biosolids (<1 HE/L or gram of dry solids, respectively). In some cases, these levels are not easy to achieve, considering the high concentrations occurring in developing countries. Helminth eggs are associated with solid particles in wastewater, either because they behave in the same way or they are part of aggregated solids. As a result, processes related to solids removal (e.g., sedimentation, filtration, or coagulation-flocculation) will also remove most of the helminth eggs contained in wastewater. Once separated, they will concentrate in sludge where they need to be inactivated before the sludge is reused or disposed of. For this purpose, processes that increase temperature and/or pH, reduce sludge humidity, as well as the use of certain chemicals (e.g., lime, organic acids, or ammonia) achieve high inactivation (>90%). Within conventional sludge treatment methods, the use of quicklime has proven effective where high concentrations occur. However, in developing countries where high concentrations of helminth eggs are found, there is still a need for economic yet efficient inactivation methods.

In order to demonstrate that these processes meet the strict limits established by regulations and guidelines, adequate methods for identification and quantification are required. Current analytical techniques to quantify helminth eggs in environmental samples are usually time-consuming and require a high level of expertise to differentiate between species. Promising alternative methods are being developed, including the use of molecular tools as well as image processing technologies that could improve sensitivity and reduce processing time. Further validation will prove their applicability under different laboratory and/or field conditions.

Quantitative microbial risk assessment has been used to predict the human health risks from exposure to *Ascaris* eggs. Some QMRA applications suggest that helminth egg limits estimated may be initial targets and may be included in national regulations (wastewater and sludge for agricultural reuse), even though they may be less strict than those proposed by WHO and US EPA, but still they will gradually reduce infection risks from these parasites. Moreover, several QMRA results have demonstrated that additional interventions and behavior changes may be implemented to reduce the risks to acceptable levels. Nonetheless, more high-quality data is needed to improve the evaluation of different exposure scenarios and to reduce uncertainties in risk estimates.

From the point of view of environmental engineering, helminth eggs are relevant since they need to be removed from wastewater and inactivated once in sludge to break their life cycle. However, to further improve public health, other strategic measures, such as preventive chemical treatment, and specific agricultural practices, must be implemented, and thus, a multidisciplinary approach is needed to address this global problem.

Author details

Blanca Jiménez, Catalina Maya, José A. Barrios* and Inés Navarro

*Address all correspondence to: jbarriosp@iingen.unam.mx

Institute of Engineering, UNAM, Mexico, D.F., Mexico

References

[1] Navarro I, Chávez A, Maya C, Becerril E, Barrios JA, Lucario S, Jimenez B. Wastewater reuse for irrigation. In: Muhammad Salik Javaid, editor. Practices, Safe Reuse and Perspectives, Irrigation and Drainage—Sustainable Strategies and Systems. Rijeka, Croatia: InTech; 2015.

[2] Jiménez B. Irrigation in developing countries using wastewater. International Review for Environmental Strategies 2006;6(2):229–250. ISBN/ISSN: 1345-7594.

[3] World Health Organization, editor. Guidelines for the Safe Use of Wastewater, Excreta and Greywater. Vol. 2. Wastewater Use in Agriculture World Health Organization. Geneva, Switzerland; 2006. 196p. ISBN: 92-4-154683-2.

[4] Maya C, Torner-Morales FJ, Lucario ES, Hernández E, Jiménez B. Viability of six of larval and non-larval helminth eggs for different conditions of temperature, pH and dryness. Water Research 2012;46:4770–4782. doi:10.1016/j.watres.2012.06.014. ISSN: 0043-1354.

[5] Jiménez B, Maya C, Velásquez G, Torner F, Arambula F, Barrios JA, Velasco M. Identification and quantification of pathogenic helminth eggs using a digital image system. Experimental Parasitology 2016;166:164–172. doi:10.1016/j.exppara.2016.04.016.

[6] World Health Organization, editor. Guidelines for the Safe Use of Wastewater, Excreta And Greywater. Vol. 1. Policy and Regulatory Aspects. Geneva, Switzerland; World Health Organization; 2006. 100 p. ISBN:92-4-154682-4.

[7] Bogitsh BJ, Carter CE, Oeltmann TN. Blood and tissue nematodes. In: Elsevier (ed.) Human Parasitology. UK: Academic Press; 2013. pp. 329–345. ISBN: 978-0-12-415915-0.

[8] Mascarini-Serra L. Prevention of soil-transmitted helminth infection. Journal of Global Infectious Diseases 2011;3(2):175–182. doi:10.4103/0974-777X.81696.

[9] Vercruysse J, Levecke B, Prichard R. Human soil-transmitted helminths: implications of mass drug administration. Current Opinion on Infectious Diseases 2012;25:703–708. ISSN: 0951-7375.

[10] Strunz EC. Water, sanitation, hygiene, and soil-transmitted helminth infection: a systematic review and meta-analysis. PLOS Medicine 2014;11:e1001620. doi:10.1371/journal.pmed.1001620.

[11] World Health Organization, editor. Helminth Control in School-Age Children: A Guide for Managers of Control Programs. Geneva, Switzerland; World Health Organization; 2011. 75 p. ISBN: 978924154826–7.

[12] World Health Organization, editor. Eliminating Soil-Transmitted Helminthiasis as a Public Health Problem in Children: Progress Report 2001–2010 and Strategic Plan 2011–2020.Geneva, Switzerland; World Health Organization; 2012. 79 p. ISBN: 97592 4150312-9.

[13] Feachem, RG.; Bradley, DJ.; Garelick, H; Mara, D. Sanitation and disease : health aspects of excreta and wastewater management. World Bank studies in water supply and sanitation; no. 3. NY: John Wiley & Sons.

[14] Ellis K, Rodrigues P, Gomez C. Parasite ova and cysts in waste stabilization ponds. Water Research 1993;27(9):1455–1460. doi:10.1016/0043-1354(93)90025-D.

[15] Alouini Z, Jemli M. Destruction of helminth eggs by photosensitized porphyrin. Journal Environmental Monitoring 2001;3:548–551. doi:10.1039/B103471P.

[16] Silva de NR, Chan MS, Bundy AP. Morbidity and mortality due to ascariasis: re-estimation and sensitivity analysis of global numbers at risk. Tropical Medicine and International Health 1997;2(6):519–528. ISSN: 13602276.

[17] Jiménez B, Maya C, Sánchez E, Romero A, Lira L, Barrios JA. Comparison of the quantity and quality of the microbiological content of sludge in countries with low and high content of pathogens. Water Science and Technology 2002;46(10):17–24. ISSN: 0273-1223.

[18] Strauss M, Drescher S, Zurbrügg CH, Montangero A. Co-composting of faecal sludge and municipal organic waste. A Literature and State-of-Knowledge Review. Dübendorf, Switzerland: Swiss Federal Institute of Environmental Science and Technology (EAWAG) and IMWI; 2003.

[19] Jimenez B, Austin A, Cloete E, Phasha C. Using Ecosan sludge for crop production. Water Science and Technology 2006;5(54):169–177. ISSN: 0273-1223.

[20] Jiménez B, Wang L. Sludge treatment and management. Chap. 10. In: Ujang Z, Henze M (eds.) Municipal Wastewater Management in Developing Countries: Principles and Engineering. London, UK: IWA Publishing; 2006. pp. 237–292. ISBN: 1-84339-030-2.

[21] Thomas-Soccol V, Paulino RC, Castro EA. Metodologia para análise parasilógica em lodo de esgoto (Methodology for parasitological analysis of sewage sludge). In: Andreoli, Bonnet (eds.). Manual de métodos para análises microbiológicas e parasitológica em reciclagem agrícola de lodo de esgoto (Handbook of microbial and parasitological methods for agricultural recycling of sewage sludge). Curitiva, Brazil; 2000. 28–41 (Portuguese).

[22] McGarry MG, Stainforth J. Compost, Fertilizer and Biogas Production from Human and Farm Wastes in the Peoples' Republic of China. Ontario, Canada: International Development Research Centre (IDRC) Ottawa; 1978. 94 pp. ISSN: 0889361401.

[23] Stott R, Jenkins T, Shabana M, May E. A survey of the microbial quality of wastewater in Ismailia, Egypt and the Implications for wastewater reuse. Water Science and Technology 1997;35(11–12):211–217. doi:10.1016/S0273-1223(97)00261-8.

[24] Hall J. Sludge management in developing countries. In: Lowe P, Hudson JA (eds.) Proceedings of the Joint CIWEM, 5th European Biosolids and Organic Residuals Conference Seminar 1, Paper 3. November 2000, Wakefield, UK. Aqua Enviro Consultancy Services; 2000.

[25] Sudo R, Aiba S. Advances in water pollution research. In: Jaag O, Baars JK, Pearson EA. (eds.) Proceedings: 2nd International Conference, August 1964, Tokyo, Japan. Oxford: Pergamon Press; 1964. pp. 282–284. doi: 10.1002/iroh.19670520415

[26] Schwartzbrod J, Stien JL, Bouhoum K, Baleux B. Impact of wastewater treatment on helminth eggs. Water Sciences and Technology 1989;21(3):295–297.

[27] Chale-Matsau JRB. Persistence of human pathogens in a crop grown from sewage sludge treated soil. PhD thesis. Faculty of Engineering, University of Pretoria, Pretoria; 2005.

[28] Pillay S, Foxon K, Rodda N, Smith M, Buckley C. The use of effluent from an anaerobic baffled reactor (ABR) for irrigation in a peri-urban community. In: Ecosan GTZ (ed.) 3rd International Ecological Sanitation Conference. Durban, South Africa: DFID, EcoSanRes, CSIR; 2005. pp. 445–449.

[29] Bradby RM, Hadidy S. Parasitic infestation and the use of untreated sewage for irrigation of vegetables with particular reference to Aleppo, Syria. Public Health Engineer 1981;9: 154–157.

[30] Stoll N. This wormy world. Journal of Parasitology 1947;33(1):1–43.

[31] Jiménez B, Maya C, Galván M. Helminth ova control in wastewater and sludge for advanced and conventional sanitation. Water Science and Technology 2007;56(5):43–51. doi:10.2166/wst.2007.555.

[32] Gaspard P, Wiart J, Schwartzbrod J. Parasitological contamination of urban sludge used for agricultural purposes. Waste Management and Research 1997;14:429–436. doi: 10.1006/wmre.1996.0097.

[33] Jiménez B, Maya C, Salgado G. The elimination of helminth ova, faecal coliforms, Salmonella and protozoan cysts by various physicochemical processes in wastewater and sludge. Water Science and Technology 2001;43(12):179–182. ISSN: 0273-1223.

[34] Pullan RL, Smith JL, Jasrasaria R, Brooker SJ. Global numbers of infection and disease burden of soil transmitted helminth infections in 2010. Parasites and Vectors. 2014;7(1): 37. ISSN: 1756-3305. http://researcholine.lshtm.ac.uk/1496142/

[35] Brown HW, Belding LD. Parasitología Clínica. Interamericana, Buenos Aires: S.A.; 1965 (Spanish).

[36] Wharton DA. Nematode egg-shells. Parasitology 1980;81:447–463. doi:10.1017/S003118200005616X.

[37] Fairweather I, Threadgold LT. *Hymenolepis nana*: the fine structure of the embryonic envelopes. Parasitology 1981;82:429–443. doi:10.1017/S0031182000066968.

[38] Lýsek H, Malínský J, Janisch R. Ultrastructure of eggs of *Ascaris lumbricoides* Linneaeus, 1758 I. Egg-shells. Folia Parasitologica 1985;32:381–384. ISSN: 1803-6465.

[39] Quilès F, Balandier JY, Capizzi-Banas S. In situ characterization of a microorganism surface by Raman microspectroscopy: the shell of *Ascaris* eggs. Analytical and Bioanalytical Chemistry 2006;386:249–255. doi:10.1007/s00216-006-0638-4.

[40] Barret J. Studies on the induction of permeability in *Ascaris lumbricoides* eggs. Parasitology 1976;73(1):109–121. PMID: 987567.

[41] Clarke AJ, Perry RN. The induction of permeability in egg shells of *Ascaris* suum prior to hatching. International Journal for Parasitology 1988;18(7):987–990. doi: 10.1016/0020-7519(88)90182-8.

[42] Vos T, et al. Global, regional, and national incidence, prevalence, and years lived with disability for 301 acute and chronic diseases and injuries in 188 countries, 1990–2013: a systematic analysis for the Global Burden of Disease Study 2013. The Lancet 2015;386(9995):743–800. doi:10.1016/S0140-6736(15)60692-4.

[43] Kassai T, Cordero del Campillo M, Euzeby J, Gaafar S, Hiepe T, Himonas CA. Standardized nomenclature of animal parasitic diseases (SNOAPAD). Veterinarian Parasitology 1988;29:299–326. doi:10.1016/0304-4017(88)90148-3.

[44] World Health Organization, editor. Health Guidelines for the Use of Wastewater in Agriculture and Aquaculture, Technical Report Series No. 778. Geneva, Switzerland; World Health Organization;1989. ISBN: 924120778-7.

[45] Asano T, editor. Wastewater Reclamation and Reuse: Water Quality Management Library. Vol. 10. Lancaster, Pennsylvania, USA: Techonomic Publishing Inc.; 1998. doi: 10.5772/59361.

[46] Cotruvo J. Water Reclamation and Groundwater Recharge in the USA Ongoing and Planned Water Reuse Related Project in EU and Mediterranean countries. WHO Expert Consultation on Health Risks in Aquifer Recharge by Reclaimed Water. Budapest; 2001.

[47] Dillon P, Toze S, Pavelic P. Australian water quality guidelines and research on subsurface storage of reclaimed water Ongoing and Planned Water Reuse Related Project in EU and Mediterranean Countries. WHO Expert Consultation on Health Risks in Aquifer Recharge by Reclaimed Water. Budapest; 2001.

[48] US Environmental Protection Agency. Part 503—Standards for the Use and Disposal of Sewage Sludge. Rules and Regulations. Federal Register 1993;58(32):9248–9415.

[49] US Environmental Protection Agency. A Guide to the Biosolids Risk Assessment for the EPA Part 503 Rule. Washington, DC, USA: Environmental Protection Agency; 1995.

[50] Tellez A, Morales W, Rivera T, Meyer E, Leiva B, Linder E. Prevalence of intestinal parasites in the human population of León, Nicaragua. Acta Tropica 1997;66:119–125. doi:10.1016/S0001-706X(97)00037-5.

[51] Howard SC, Donnelly CA, Kabatereine NB, Ratard RC, Brooker S. Spatial and intensity-dependent variations in associations between multiple species Helminth infections. Acta Tropica 2002;83:141–149. doi:10.1016/S0001-706X(02)00093-1.

[52] Berhe N, Madhin G, Erko B, Smith T, Gedamu S, Bereded D, Moore R, Habte E, Redda A, Gebre-Michael T, Gundersen SG. Variations in helminth faecal egg counts in Kato-Katz thick smears and their implications in assessing infection status with *Schistosoma mansoni*. Acta Tropica 2004;92:205–212. doi:10.1016/jactatropica.2003.06.011.

[53] Regli S, Rose JB, Haas CN, Gerba CP. Modeling risk from Giardia and viruses in drinking water. American Water Works Association Journal 1991;83(11):76–84.

[54] Rose JB, Haas CN, Regli S. Risk assessment and control of waterborne Giardiasis. American Journal of Public Health 1991;81(6):709–713. doi:10.2105/AJPH.81.6.709.

[55] Haas CN, Rose JB, Gerba CP. Quantitative Microbial Risk Assessment. New York: Wiley; 1999.

[56] Crockett CS, Haas CN, Fazil A, Rose JB, Gerba CP. Prevalence of shigellosis in the U.S.: consistency with dose-response information. International Journal of Food Microbiology 1996;30(1–2):87–100.

[57] Fazil AM. A Quantitative Risk Assessment Model for Salmonella. M.S. Thesis, Drexel University, Philadelphia, PA, USA; 1996.

[58] Medema GJ, Teunis PF, Havelaar AH, Haas CN. Assessment of the dose-response relationship of Campylobacter jejuni. International Journal of Food Microbiology 1996;30(1–2):101–111. doi:10.1016/0168-1605(96)00994-4.

[59] Teunis PF, Nagelkerke NJ, Haas CN. Dose response models for infectious gastroenteritis. Risk Analysis 1999;19(6):1251–1260.

[60] Navarro I, Jimenez B, Cifuentes E, Lucario S. Application of helminth ova infection dose curve to estimate the risks associated with biosolid application on soil. Journal of Water and Health 2009;7(1):31–44. doi:10.2166/wh.2009.113.

[61] Haas CN. Microbial dose response modeling: past, present & future. Environmental Science and Technology 2014;49(3):1245–1259. doi:10.1021/es504422q.

[62] Navarro I, Jiménez B. Evaluation of the WHO helminth eggs criteria using a QMRA approach for the safe reuse of wastewater and sludge in developing countries. Water Science and Technology 2011;63(7):1499–1505. doi:10.2166/wst.2011.394. ISSN: 0273-1223. ISSN: 0273-1223.

[63] Mara D, Hamilton AJ, Sleigh A, Karavarsamis N. Tools for risk analysis: updating the 2006 WHO guidelines. In: Dreschsel P, Scott CA, Raschild-Sally L, Redwood M, Bahri A (eds.) Wastewater Irrigation and Health: Assessing and Mitigating Risks in Low-Income Countries. London: Earthscan; 2010. pp. 89–100.

[64] Mara D, Sleigh A. Estimation of norovirus and *Ascaris* infection risks to urban farmers in developing countries using wastewater for crop irrigation. Journal of Water and Health 2010;8(3):572–576.

[65] Ayres RM, Stott R, Mara DD, Lee DL. Wastewater reuse in agriculture and the risk of intestinal nematode infection. Parasitologica Today 1992;8(1):32–35. doi:10.1016/0169-4758(92)90309-P.

[66] Ensink JHJ, van der Hoek W. Implementation of the WHO guidelines for the safe use of wastewater in Pakistan: balancing risks and benefits. Journal of Water Health 2009;7(3):464–468.

[67] Williams DL, Pepper IL, Gerba CP. Survival of *Ascaris* ova in desert soils: a risk assessment. Journal of Residuals Science and Technology 2012;9(4):151–157. doi: 10.2166/wh.2009.061.

[68] Seidu R, Sjølander I, Abubakari A, Amoah D, Larbi JA, Stenström TA. Modeling the die-off of *E. coli* and *Ascaris* in wastewater irrigated vegetables: implications for microbial health risk reduction associated with irrigation cessation. Water Science and Technology 2013;68(5):1013–1021. doi:10.2166/wst.2013.335.

[69] Barker SF, Amoah P, Drechsel P. A probabilistic model of gastroenteritis risks associated with consumption of street food salads in Kumasi, Ghana: Evaluation of methods to estimate pathogen dose from water, produce or food quality. Science of the Total Environment 2014;487(1):130–142. doi:10.1016/j.scitotenv.2014.03.108.

[70] Kundu A, Poma HR, Jenkins MW, Rajal VB, Wuertz S. QMRA of intestinal nematode infection via multimedia exposure pathways. In: Proceedings 7th International Congress on Environmental Modelling and Software: Bold Visions for Environmental Modeling, IEMSs 2014; vol. 3. pp. 1482–1491.

[71] Jiménez B, Barrios JA, Maya C. Class B biosolids production from wastewater sludge with high pathogenic content generated in an advanced primary treatment. Water Science and Technology 2000;42(9):103–110. ISSN: 0273-1223.

[72] Mara D. Domestic Wastewater Treatment in Developing Countries. London: Earth Scan; 2003.

[73] Jiménez B. Helminth ova removal from wastewater for agriculture and aquaculture reuse. Water Science and Technology 2007;55(1–2):485–493. ISSN: 0273-1223.

[74] Chavez A, Jimenez B, Maya C. Particle size distribution as a useful tool for microbial detection, Water Science and Technology 2004;50(2):179–186. ISSN: 0273-1223.

[75] Landa H, Capella A, Jiménez B. Particle size distribution in an effluent from an advanced primary treatment and its removal during filtration. Water Science and Technology 1997;36(4):159–165. doi:10.1016/S0273-1223(97)00435-6.

[76] Jimenez B, Chavez A. Low cost technology for reliable use of Mexico city's wastewater for agricultural irrigation. Environmental Technology 2002;9(1–2):95–108. doi:10.1016/j.resconrec.2009.08.002.

[77] Brix H. Chapter 2: wastewater treatment in constructed wetlands: system design, removal process and treatment performance. In: Moshiri G (eds.) Constructed Wetlands for Water Quality Improvement. USA: CRC Press; 1993. pp. 9–22.

[78] Olguin EJ, Hernandez E. Use of aquatic plants for recovery of nutrients and heavy metals from wastewater. Inter-America program for environmental technology cooperation in the key industry sector. Roundtable on Municipal Water 15–17 Mars 1998, Vancouver Canada. http:/www.idrc.ca/industry/canada_el4html.

[79] Rivera F, Warren A, Curds CR, Robles E, Gutierrez A, Gallegos E, Calderon A. The application on the root zone method for the treatment and reuse of high-strength abattoir waste in Mexico. Water Science and Technology 1997;35(5):271–278.

[80] Stott R, Jenkins T, Baghat M, Shalaby I. Capacity of constructed wetlands to remove parasite eggs from wastewater in Egypt. Water Science and Technology 1999;40(3): 117–123. PII: SO273-1223(99)00454-0.

[81] Krasnonos LI. Many-years viability of *Ascaris* eggs (*Ascaris lumbricoides*) in soil of Samarkand. Medicine and Parasitology 1978;47:103–106. (Abstract in: Trop. Dis. Bull. 1978;75(10):991–992).

[82] Popat SC, Yates MV, Deshusses MA. Kinetics of inactivation of indicator pathogens during thermophilic anaerobic digestion. Water Research 2010;44:5965–5972. doi: 10.1016/j.watres.2010.07.045.

[83] Kato S, Fogarty E, Bowman DD. Effect of aerobic and anaerobic digestion on the viability of *Cryptosporidium parvum* oocysts and *Ascaris* suum eggs. International Journal Environmental Health Research 2003;13:169–179. doi:10.1080/096031203100 0098071.

[84] Gantzer C, Gaspard P, Galvez L, Huyard A, Dumouthier N, Schwartzbrod J. Monitoring of bacterial and parasitological contamination during various treatment of sludge. Water Research 2001;35 3763–3770. doi:10.1016/S0043-1354(01)00105-1. 12230157

[85] Capizzi-Banas S, Schwartzbrod J. Irradiation of *Ascaris* ova in sludge using an electron beam accelerator. Water Research 2001;135:2256–2260. doi:10.1016/S0043-1354(00) 00503-0.

[86] Johnson PW, Dixon R, Ross AD. An in-vitro test for assessing the viability of *Ascaris* suum eggs exposed to various sewage treatment processes. International Journal Parasitology 1998;28:627–633.

[87] Méndez JM, Jiménez BE, Barrios JA. Improved alkaline stabilization of municipal wastewater sludge. Water Science and Technology 2002;46(10):139–146. ISSN: 0273–1223.

[88] Ghiglietti R, Gench C, Mateo L, Calcaterra E, Colombi A. Survival of *Ascaris* suum in amonia treated wasterwater sludge. Bioresource Technology 1998;59:195–198.

[89] Barrios J, Jiménez B, Maya C. Treatment of sludge with peracetic acid to reduce the microbial content. Journal of Residuals Science and Technology 2004;1(1):69–74. ISSN: 1544-8053.

[90] Aguilar P, Jiménez B, Maya C, Orta T, Luna V. Disinfection of sludge with high pathogenic content using silver and other compounds. Water Science and Technology 2006;54(5):179–187. doi:10.2166/wst.2006.561. ISSN: 0273-1223.

[91] Bowman DD, Little MD, Reimers RS. Precision and accuracy of an assay for detecting *Ascaris* eggs in various biosolid matrices. Water Research 2003;37:2063–2072. doi: 10.1016/S0043-1354(02)00597-3.

[92] Gyawali P, Ahmed W, Jagals P, Sidhu JPS, Toze S. Comparison of concentration methods for rapid detection of hookworm ova in wastewater matrices using quantitative PCR. Experimental Parasitology 2015;159:160–167. doi:10.1016/j.exppara.2015.09.002.

[93] Gyawali P, Sidhu JPS, Ahmed W, Jagals P, Toze S. Rapid concentration and sensitive detection of hookworm ova from wastewater matrices using a real-time PCR method. Experimental Parasitology 2015;159:5–12. doi:10.1016/j.exppara.2015.08.009.

[94] Raynal M, Villegas EN, Nelson KL. Enumeration of viable and non-viable larvated *Ascaris* eggs with quantitative PCR. Journal of Water and Health 2012;10:594–604. doi: 10.2166/wh.2012.101.

[95] Pecson BM, Barrios JA, Johnson DR, Nelson KL. A real-time PCR method for quantifying viable *Ascaris* eggs using the first internally transcribed spacer region of ribosomal DNA. Applied and Environmental Microbiology 2006;72:7864–7872. doi:10.1128/AEM.01983-06.

Section 3

Interactions with Associated Diseases

Chapter 4

Helminthiasis: A Systematic Review of the Immune Interactions Present in Individuals Coinfected with HIV and/or Tuberculosis

Zilungile L. Mkhize-Kwitshana,
Rebecca Tadokera and Musawenkosi H.L. Mabaso

Additional information is available at the end of the chapter

http://dx.doi.org/10.5772/106429

Abstract

Helminth infections are highly endemic in parts of the world where the two killer epidemics caused by *Mycobacterium tuberculosis* (*M.tb*) and the human immunodeficiency virus (HIV) intersect. Sub-Saharan Africa is hardest hit by this epidemiological overlap. Consequently, several studies have investigated the immunological outcomes of helminth coinfection with either HIV or *M.tb*, to elucidate the central hypothesis that chronic infection with helminths exacerbates the course of HIV and tuberculosis disease. However, there is no conclusive evidence to confirm whether helminth-induced immunity modulates HIV- and TB-specific immune responses and their pathogenesis or vice versa. The present chapter summarizes the epidemiology, clinical course, and immune interactions during helminths and HIV/TB coinfections and undertakes a systematic review of the existing literature published from Africa on this subject. The aim was to determine if chronic helminthiasis has a negative impact on HIV and TB infections. A PubMed search was undertaken with no language and time restrictions. Search terms used included a varied combination of "Helminth coinfection and immunity and TB coinfection or TB immunity and HIV coinfection or HIV immunity and Africa." Names of individual species were also permutated in the search terms. Reviews and bibliographies of selected articles were screened to identify additional relevant articles or studies. Of the total 1021 articles retrieved, 47 were relevant with 31 helminth and HIV coinfection and 16 helminths and TB coinfection articles. While many studies failed to find a negative impact of helminth infection on immune responses to HIV and/or TB, a significant number found evidence of deleterious effects of coinfection with helminths such as immune activation, impaired Th1 responses to TB antigens, higher viral loads, lower CD4+ counts, and increased risks of antiretroviral immunologic failure, mother to child HIV transmission or TB disease. Some of the helminth-induced immune dysregulation was reversed by deworming, while some studies found no benefit of antihelminthic treatment. More studies particularly in Southern Africa are needed to increase the much sought evidence of the impact of deworming among HIV-infected individuals as this seems the most feasible, cost-effective intervention with little or no serious adverse effects. Lastly, with the expansion of ART and increased access to HIV treatment, the effects of helminths on vaccines, TB, and antiretroviral treatments efficacy also need serious consideration, in light of the suggestive evidence of possible immunologic failure due to helminth coinfection.

Keywords: helminths, *Mycobacterium tuberculosis*, human immunodeficiency virus, co-infection, immune-response, Africa

1. Introduction

1.1. Overview

Helminthiasis is an infection with either flukes (trematodes), tapeworms (cestodes), or roundworms (nematodes) [1]. These worms are highly endemic in parts of the world where the two killer epidemics caused by *Mycobacterium tuberculosis* (*M.tb*) and the human immunodeficiency virus (HIV) intersect [2]. This epidemiological overlap between helminthic infections, TB and HIV, is more common in lower and middle-income countries, particularly sub-Saharan Africa (SSA). This is one of the hardest hit regions with regards to HIV and tuberculosis [2], while helminth infections are also highly endemic in this part of the world [3]. Almost 70% of the population infected with HIV resides in SSA, which also carries two-thirds of the global burden of helminthiasis [2, 3]. Regrettably, helminth infections as part of the neglected tropical diseases (NTDs) are still largely neglected and not a prioritized research domain in most regions where they are highly prevalent and overlap with HIV and *M.tb*. This raises important research questions about the public health implications of helminth coinfection with HIV and/or *M.tb* in terms of pathogenesis and treatment outcomes of all these diseases. Furthermore, although individual helminth-, HIV-, and *M.tb*-specific immune responses have been extensively investigated [2], the precise immune correlates of protection remain mostly unknown.

Several studies have investigated the immunological aspects of helminth coinfection with either HIV or *M.tb*, to elucidate the central hypothesis that chronic infection with helminths exacerbates the course of HIV and tuberculosis disease [2]. Owing to the complexity of the interaction at molecular, cellular, and humoral levels, the differences in study designs resulting from financial and ethical challenges of properly designed randomized control trials for such studies, many of these investigations have reported inconclusive or contradictory results. As a result, to date, there is no conclusive evidence to confirm whether helminth-induced immunity modulates HIV- and TB-specific immune responses and their pathogenesis or vice versa.

There is a need therefore to constantly explore the work on the immunological consequences of dual infections in order to condense and update this knowledge for policy makers in terms of a holistic management of coinfections in areas where all these infections are coendemic. The present chapter aims to review published research on the immune interactions during coinfection with helminths, HIV, and *M.tb* in the African region, a continent with a very high burden of all three infectious diseases. A brief description of the epidemiology, clinical course, and immune interactions during helminths and HIV/TB coinfections is given and then followed by a systematic review of the existing literature on this subject.

1.2. Epidemiology of helminthiasis

More than 2 billion people worldwide are infected with helminths including geohelminths or soil-transmitted helminths, schistosomes, and filarial worms, the vast majority of whom are in low-/medium-income countries. Individuals who are affected frequently harbor more than one species of worm at a time [4]. The major human helminth species of public health importance include *Ascaris, Trichuris, Hookworms* (*Necator americanus, Ancylostoma duodenale*), *Trichinella, Filaria, Onchocercaria, Ecchinococcus, Enterobius, Strongyloides, Taenia,* and *Schistosoma* species. It has been estimated that schistosomiasis and soil-transmitted helminths (sTH) together account for 40% of all the tropical disease burden excluding malaria and that infectious and parasitic diseases are the primary causes of death worldwide [5, 6].

Soil-transmitted helminths alone constitute the highest burden. Globally, an estimated 438.9 million people (95% confidence interval (CI), 406.3–480.2 million) were reported to be infected with hookworm in 2010, 819.0 million (95% CI, 771.7–891.6 million) with *A. lumbricoides*, and 464.6 million (95% CI, 429.6–508.0 million) with *T. trichiura* [6]. In underdeveloped regions, geohelminths cycle via pollution of the soil by feces containing worm ova or eggs from infested humans. Individuals get infected through ingesting eggs in undercooked, unwashed, and unpeeled fruits and vegetables, in contaminated water sources, or eggs ingested by children who play in the contaminated soil and then put their hands in their mouths without washing them. In hookworm infections, eggs hatch in the soil, releasing larvae which penetrate the skin of people walking barefoot on the contaminated soil. In the case of schistosomes, water is polluted by urine and/or feces [4]. These epidemiological cycles have been exacerbated because of overcrowding in densely populated informal settlements without adequate sanitation or clean water, owing to rapid urbanization and migration. Transmission is therefore directly linked to availability of clean water supplies, poor hygiene, inadequate sanitation, the presence of infective worm eggs in the environment, and climatic factors. In other developing countries such as Central America and the Caribbean and parts of East and Southeast Asia, socioeconomic and sanitation improvements and rollout of large-scale regular deworming programs have reduced the previously high infection rates. In Central and Southern Asia, large numbers of helminth infections still occur in certain regions owing to variations in environmental and socioeconomic conditions, while in South America helminthiasis is distributed in pockets of poverty-stricken indigenous populations. In the Middle East, transmission is limited by hot and dry weather but high prevalence is still found in areas with suitable climate within informal settlements [3]. In developed countries, the general availability of efficacious deworming drugs, clean water, and effective sanitation has eliminated most of these parasites such that more serious infections do not occur in these regions and mostly minor or imported cases are reported [7].

In general, helminths develop through three stages: eggs, larva, and adult worms, which determine both their epidemiology and pathogenesis in humans [8]. An example is illustrated in the case of soil-transmitted helminths where the eggs have a 3-week maturation stage in the soil that requires temperate, moist, and humid soil before they become infective [4]. Subsequently, these worms are most prevalent in regions with tropical and subtropical climate. In terms of the pathogenesis, larvae and eventually adult worms may cause direct pathology through migration, metabolic activity, or blockage and damage to the internal organs they finally parasitize.

1.3. Epidemiology of HIV

Globally, 36.7 million [34.0–39.8 million] people were living with HIV at the end of 2015 [9]. During the 35 years of the epidemic, more than 70 million people have been infected with HIV globally and about 35 million people have died [10]. The distribution of the HIV infection varies dramatically from region to region. Globally, sub-Saharan Africa is the most severely affected, with nearly 70% of the people living with HIV worldwide being from the region. At least one in every 25 adults (4.4%) in this region is living with HIV [10]. The data as at the end of 2014 is summarized in **Table 1** and illustrates the skewed distribution of the HIV virus across the globe [11]. The sub-Saharan region has consistently been carrying the heaviest burden of the HIV infection globally.

Region	Number of people living with HIV in 2014
Sub-Saharan Africa	25.8 million
Asia and the Pacific	5 million
Western and Central Europe and North America	2.4 million
Latin America	1.7 million
Eastern Europe and Central Asia	1.5 million
Middle East and North Africa	280,000
The Caribbean	240,000

Adapted from UNAIDS data http://www.avert.org/global-hiv-and-aids-statistics [11].

Table 1. Global distribution of HIV infection (2014).

1.4. Epidemiology of *Mycobacterium tuberculosis*

Tuberculosis (TB) remains a major global public health problem and ranks second only to HIV as a cause of death worldwide [12]. TB is an infectious disease caused by the bacillus *Mycobacterium tuberculosis* (*M.tb*). It typically affects the lungs (pulmonary TB) but can disseminate to affect other sites as well (extra pulmonary TB). The disease is spread in the air when people who have pulmonary TB disease expel bacteria, for example, by coughing. It is estimated that a third of the world's population is infected with *M.tb*. In 2015, the World Health Organization reported 9 million TB cases with 1.5 million deaths annually [13]. Furthermore, according to the WHO, the African region has more than 24% of the world's TB cases and deaths, while approximately 78% of total TB deaths and 73% of TB deaths among HIV-negative people occurred in the African and the Southeast Asian regions combined [13]. On a global scale, the African region alone accounts for at least 80% of TB cases dually infected with HIV worldwide. This is because in many African countries, the tuberculosis and HIV epidemics are fueling each other.

In general, a relatively small proportion of the estimated 2–3 billion people infected with *M.tb* globally will develop TB disease during their lifetime (approximately 10%) [14]. This is because although healthy people often will get infected by the bacilli, they are usually able to fight it off or keep it under control to a large extent. Other people may only succumb to TB disease years later, often when the immune system has been weakened by conditions such as HIV infection, resulting in the reactivation of latent subclinical *M.tb* infection. Thus, it has been established that the two categories of people developing TB disease include (i) those who have been infected with TB bacilli and (ii) persons with compromised immune systems, possibly due to other health conditions. Among the latter, HIV, diabetes, silicosis, low body weight, and certain medical treatments, among others, have been established as known risk factors for the development of TB disease.

Important factors in the management of TB include early detection, treatment, and management of infected individuals in order to curb unabated transmission of this air-borne infection. Detection and treatment relies heavily on the diagnostic capacity and linkage to care. To date, the most widely used method for diagnosing TB worldwide remains sputum smear microscopy, in which bacteria are observed in sputum samples examined under a microscope, a method which was developed over 100 years ago. However, in countries with more developed laboratory capacity, the cases of TB are also diagnosed via the culture method which is currently the gold standard in TB diagnostics. Technological advancements in the last few years have resulted in the use of rapid molecular tests to diagnose TB. Use of these techniques, such as the GeneXpert, is now on the increase, with some countries now gradually phasing out the use of smear microscopy for TB diagnosis [15].

TB is a poverty-related disease. As such, the financial demands of proper diagnosis using laboratory techniques are juxtaposed by the limited resources in poor regions, and the financial deprivation among the poor hinder optimum access to health care facilities. These factors imply that a significant proportion of TB patients remains either unrecognized and untreated or not notified, thus exacerbating transmission. Without treatment, the natural cycle of TB infection is that a person deteriorates progressively, with the term "consumption" having been used in the old days to describe the disease. The death rate in untreated TB cases is very high. Studies from the prechemotherapy era showed that at least 70% of people who had microbiologically confirmed TB died within 10 years of the infection. Currently, the effective chemotherapeutic management of normal drug-sensitive TB lasts for at least 6–9 months. This long treatment duration, coupled with side effects of anti-TB drugs, leads to noncompliance resulting in the emergence of drug-resistant TB in recent years [15]. The treatment of drug-resistant TB is much more complicated requiring much longer treatment regimens of up to 2 years, an even so, with very poor prognosis and suboptimum treatment outcomes. Treatment outcomes therefore also bear a direct impact on the epidemiology of tuberculosis.

1.5. Clinical course and immune responses during helminthiasis and HIV coinfection

Helminthiasis can be due to infection with a wide range of species which occupy a variety of niches within the human body ranging from intestinal lumen, lymphatics, intravascular, or intracellular compartments [1]. The clinical course will then differ from one species to another depending on the course of infection and maturation cycle in the host and where the adult worms eventually reside. The current work will not attempt to dissect the clinical course of each species. Broadly, the clinical course of helminthiasis is associated with their infection route and the final tissue or organ in which the adult worms reside and multiply.

Helminths have complex life cycles within the human host and undergo a series of developmental stages in different parts of the human body. These different stages result in the host being exposed to various stage-specific antigens in a range of host tissues and organs such as the skin, lungs, gut, heart, liver, bladder, and brain and pass through the circulatory and lymphatic systems [1]. Subsequently, the clinical manifestations can be associated with the early infection phases such as during the larval entry and migration such as the hookworm's ground itch skin, the perianal itch, and pruritis vulvae in enterobiasis [1]. Migrating larvae may also induce immune reactions as they pass through the tissues, such as the cutaneous syndrome as a result of hookworm penetrating the skin. Another is illustrated by the development of *Ascaris lumbricoides* after the ingested eggs have hatched in the human gastrointestinal tract [1, 8]. The larvae migrate through the blood and via the lungs where they cause an eosinophilic pneumonitis syndrome, before being coughed up and reswallowed into the intestinal tract where they establish as adult worms [1]. The worms may cause pathology directly as they migrate through organs causing tissue damage, or indirectly through the immune response they induce. A case in point is the schistosomiasis-induced inflammatory response and the pathological sequelae associated with the eggs lodged in the urogenital mucosa and organs [16].

The parasites have different lifespans, which vary from species to species, for example, adult schistosome worms can live for up to 5 years in the host in the absence of chemotherapy. *Onchocecaria volvulus* has a life expectancy of up to 8–10 years while *Ascaris lumbricoides* is 1 year. Those with a short life cycle have a faster reinfection rate after chemotherapy and are highly fecund, for example, an adult Ascaris female can produce 200,000 eggs per day [17].

Helminthiasis is also associated with a wide variety of clinical symptoms ranging from gastrointestinal (diarrhoea, vomiting, pharyngeal irritation, cough, dyspnea, hoarseness nausea, bloating, malabsorption), systemic (anemia, lymphedema, cystercercosis epileptic fits) to organ occlusion. Some infections are cleared by the host's immune response while most establish and become chronic. It is noted that clinically, many infected individuals experience minor symptoms or remain asymptomatic. Eighty percent of the heavy infections are carried by 20% of the infected population and these individuals suffer serious life-threatening disease

[17]. However, owing to the large number of infected individuals globally, this small percentage translates to large numbers of people with such morbidity. Importantly, the full-scale implications of helminthiasis even in the absence of symptoms and overt disease is the result of their subtle but deleterious impact on the other major killer pathogens such as the HIV and *M.tb* as outlined in the following sections.

1.5.1. Immune response to helminths

Although helminths comprise of a spectrum of species, a striking phenomenon found during helminthiasis is an almost universal immune response elicited by these pathogens. The response is characterized by the following archetypical features:

- Consistent induction of a strong T helper 2 (Th2) immune response by CD4+ T helper 2 cells with the production of type 2 cytokines: interleukin (IL)-4, IL-5, IL-9, IL-10, and IL-13.
- Increased levels of regulatory cells, molecules, and cytokines.
- Classic eosinophilia, increased numbers of mast cells, and basophils accompanied by very high immunoglobulin E (IgE) levels.
- Existence in the host for protracted periods, sometimes years, in the presence of strong immune responses directed against the parasites.
- The resultant chronic activation of the immune system from the persistent worm and egg or larval antigenic challenge is associated with an increased rate of programmed cell death (apoptosis).
- Induction of specific and generalized immune suppression (anergy) as one of the strategies to survive in the face of strong immune responses [2].

Early in the infection, macrophages and dendritic cells are the first line of defense in the innate immune response. These cells interact with parasite antigens and present them to T cells and also secrete type 1 and inflammatory cytokines such as interleukin (IL)-12, tumor necrosis factor alpha (TNFα), IL-6, and IL-8 [17, 18]. Other cell types such as the NK T cells in the gut mucosa secrete IL-4, promoting the differentiation of the CD4 T cells toward a Th2 phenotype [18]. These Th2 cells will secrete Th2 cytokines and also promote antibody isotype switch to IgE [18]. CD4 T cells therefore play a key role in the development of the strong Th2 adaptive immune response to helminths. Cytokines also recruit and prompt proliferation of other granulocytic cells such as eosinophils, mast cells, and basophils which mediate extracellular killing and expulsion of the worms through increased mucus secretion by goblet cells [18, 19].

A variety of mechanisms through which helminths evade the strong immune responses have been elucidated. Central among these is the increased number of regulatory cells which play a key role in dampening the immune response [2, 19]. These cells secrete the downregulatory cytokines IL-10 and transforming growth factor β (TGFβ) which in turn increases cytotoxic T lymphocyte antigen-4 (CTLA-4) expression in T cells. On the other hand, the costimulatory molecule CD28 which facilitates T-cell intracellular signaling and activation in response to antigenic stimulation is decreased during helminth infection [2]. This costimulatory molecule is essential for completion of T-cell activation after the T-cell receptor binds the antigen presented in association with the major histocompatibility complex (MHC) [18]. CTLA-4 competes with CD28 for binding in T cells, as a regulatory mechanism to prevent uncontrolled immune responses. Cells continually stimulated by parasite antigens in the absence of CD28 fail to mount an effective immune response and remain anergic [2, 18]. Increased CTLA-4 induced by chronic helminthiasis will outcompete the CD28 binding, thereby rendering the T cells partially activated and unresponsive [2].

Other mechanisms of immune diversion by helminths include secretion of decoy molecules and cytokine homologs such as the macrophage-inhibitory factor (MIF) which switches macrophages to differentiate toward a type 2 phenotype that is counter inflammatory. Helminths also secrete protease inhibitors that interfere with antigen presentation and cell proliferation [19]. These pathogens also modulate innate cells such as the dendritic cells and macrophages toward the Th2 phenotype inducing alternatively activated macrophages. The diversion and regulation of the immune response toward a favorable niche such as promoting wound healing; dampening of the inflammatory type 1 toward Th2; induction of alternatively activated macrophages that do not secrete IL-12 (which promotes the differentiation of Th1 cells); and secretion of other molecules that interact with the host tissues are all mechanisms that optimize the existence and survival of the parasites *in vivo* without causing extensive harm and possible death of the host [19, 20].

Other key cellular changes that occur during helminthiasis include decreased numbers of CD4+ and increased frequency of CD8+ cells [21], increased expression of chemokine receptors CCR5 and CXCR4 in T cells [22], and in vaginal mucosal cells [16]. Another worm-induced immunomodulatory mechanism is the selective upregulation of programed death 1 ligand, which subsequently binds to program death-1 in T cells, thus rendering them anergic and prone to increased apoptosis [2, 19].

1.5.2. Clinical course and immune response to HIV

The immune response to HIV differs among infected individuals. The course of the infection is determined by several factors such as the viral fitness or virulence, the host genetic factors such as the association of the HLA-B27, HLA-B*5701, HLA-B*5703, HLA-B*5801, and HLA-B57 alleles [23, 24], and CCR-5 mutation [25] with resistance, as well as the immune response particularly the cytokine microenvironment—with the predominance of type-1 cytokines being more favorable. The cells of the innate immune system, the NK cells, are the source of antiviral interferons secreted in the primary phase before induction of the adaptive immune responses [18]. The effective control of HIV is chiefly dependent on the development of potent HIV-specific cytotoxic T lymphocyte response (CTL) mediated by the Th1 CD8+ lymphocytes. This was aptly demonstrated in both animal models and human studies early in the advent of HIV [26–28]. The simultaneous appearance of the CTL at the point of peak viremia is followed by the decrease in viral replication and establishment of the viral set point during the early phase of the HIV infection and the association between higher numbers of CTL, viral suppression and slower decline of CD4+ cells during all phases of the HIV infection [29].

http://dx.doi.org/10.5772/106429

The development and maintenance of competent CTLs is also dependent on robust HIV-1 specific $CD4^+$ responses (particularly HIV-1 gag-specific). Paradoxically, the classic immunological characteristic of HIV disease progression is the extensive attrition of the CD4+ lymphocytes, attributed to the fact that during the HIV infection not only HIV-infected cells are affected, but uninfected bystander $CD4^+$ cells are also depleted [30]. The overall depletion of the CD4+ cells is mediated via several mechanisms, including direct cytopathic effects on infected cells, indirect bystander killing, and increased activation-induced programed cell death or apoptosis [2].

Other prominent cellular changes during HIV infection include increased numbers of CD8+ cells, which remain high throughout the infection phases. The main functions of these cells include the secretion of the antiviral Th1 cytokine, interferon gamma (IFNγ), as well as cytolytic destruction of viral-infected cells through the granzymes and perforin system [18]. The innate cells also secrete TNFα, IL-6, and IL-8. However, it has been shown that the consistently high numbers of CD8+ cells are not related to increased antiviral potency [29] and that their function wanes as the infection progresses, although the numbers remain high.

Regulatory cells also increase because of the chronic antigenic challenge and immune activation. These changes are also accompanied by increased expression on T cells, of downregulatory molecules such as the cytotoxic T lymphocyte antigen 4 (CTLA-4), and the negative regulator of T-cell activation molecule, program death 1 (PD-1), as well as decreased costimulatory molecules, particularly CD28, which plays a key role in the induction of T lymphocyte response to antigen [18]. Normally, the CTLA-4 competition with CD28 for binding down modulates the immune stimulation to prevent a pathologic runaway or uncontrolled immune response. During chronic HIV infection, this homeostasis is disturbed by higher-than-normal levels of CTLA-4 secreted by the upregulated regulatory T cells (Tregs) which also secrete high levels of IL-10 and transforming growth factor β (TGF β) [2]. The increased levels of IL-10 and TGF β are responsible for the generalized immune suppression with disease progression. Decrease in type 1 cytokines (IL-2), a lymphoproliferative cytokine and the antiviral interferon gamma (IFNγ) and ascendancy of Th2 cytokines have been associated with HIV disease progression. The total effect is inability of T cells to respond to cognate and unrelated antigens and increased programmed cell death (apoptosis) [2]. The early viremic phase of the HIV infection is also characterized by marked increases of mainly inflammatory cytokines such as IFNγ, IFNα, IL-15, IL-22 TNFα, CXCL10, and regulatory IL-10, known as the cytokine storm. These are secreted by infected $CD4^+CCR5^+$ T cells, activated dendritic cells, monocytes, macrophages, NK cells, NKT cells, and HIV-specific T cells [29].

Owing to the chronic nature of the HIV, chronic immune activation and increased levels of regulatory cells is also another striking feature of the infection. The immune activation correlates with CD4 decline and increased apoptosis [30]. HIV infection is known to stimulate B cell and antibody forming cells. In the past, owing to the rapid mutation of the virus, the protective effects of antibodies remained contentious. However, with the advancement of molecular and computational research tools, there has been recent interest in exploiting the neutralising antibodies for therapeutic vaccine development with promising results [31].

1.5.3. Immune interaction during helminth and HIV coinfection

It is recognized that during coinfection, the effects of immune modulation and regulation is bi-directional, in other words, immune response to HIV can modulate the response to helminths [32] and vice versa. However, the focus of this work is on helminthiasis, and therefore we will examine the influence of helminths on HIV and *M.tb*. Several immune mechanisms suggest that immune responses to helminths are deleterious to immune control of intracellular pathogens such as HIV. The interaction in a dually infected host may either increase susceptibility or enhance cell-cell infection and virus replication thereby indirectly increasing transmission. The key mechanisms that are proposed to drive this interaction are summarized below.

1.5.3.1. Increased viral replication and transmission

The classic induction of a strong Th2 immune response by helminths downregulates the critical Th1 CTL response required for the control of HIV. In addition, HIV has been shown to replicate more readily in Th2 cells [33]. Uncontrolled viral replication increases transmission to other hosts (high viral load) and within the same individual. Helminthiasis and HIV infection are chronic infections, with chronic immune activation being the classic feature in both infections [2]. It is known that the HIV virus hijacks the host's natural transcription process for its own replication. The transcription factor NF-Kβ, which is present in all activated cells, binds to both host DNA promoter and viral long terminal repeat sequences (LTR) which then initiates viral transcription [18]. In addition, the nuclear factor of activated T cells (NF-AT) stabilizes the postfusion HIV complex and facilitates reverse transcription of the virus [34]. Proinflammatory cytokine signaling pathways, particularly TNFα, IL-1, and IL-2, induce these transcriptional factors [18]. IL-6 also synergizes with TNFα in monocytes to enhance HIV replication [34]. Increased levels of proinflammatory cytokines such as TNFα and IL-2 are well documented in chronic helminthiasis [2, 35]. In that way, availability of increased numbers infected, activated $CD4^+$ T cells enhances viral replication.

One of the classic features of helminthiasis is increased production of immunoglobulin E (IgE). This antibody isotype has been shown to increase viral replication as shown by increased production of the HIV capsid protein 24 (p24) and viral mRNA in a culture system. The crosslinking of the cell surface molecule CD23 by IgE leads to the production of cyclic adenosine monophosphate (cAMP), nitric oxide (NO), and tumor necrosis factor-α (TNFα), which enhance viral replication and thereby accelerate progression to AIDS [36].

1.5.3.2. Increased susceptibility to HIV

Upregulation of chemokine receptor molecules (CCR5 and CXCR4) [16, 22] by helminths increases receptor molecules on CD4-positive cells, thereby increasing the numbers of HIV susceptible cells, enhancing cell-cell infection and replication of the virus. Eosinophils constitute one of the key cellular responses during helminthiasis. Activated eosinophils express CD4 molecules, and have been shown to be infectable with HIV *in vitro* [37, 38]. Their increased numbers in genital and rectal mucosa may facilitate increased virus transmission during hetero- and homosexual interaction, respectively.

Similar to HIV, helminth infections have been reported to result in the depletion of CD4+ cells [21]. This suggests that helminth-infected individuals may be more susceptible to HIV infection as the CD4+ cells are critical for both provision of help for CD8+ cell (CTL) development, type 1 cytokine secretion as well and mounting an effective immune response to antigenic challenge [18]. In addition, CD4+ cell depletion has been directly linked to immune activation [30] which is present in chronic helminthiasis.

Both helminth and HIV infections are accompanied by increased regulatory cell networks. This results in a high degree of reduced capacity to respond to cognate and bystander (unrelated) antigen stimulation. The chronic immune activation is also associated with increased apoptosis and rapid cell turnover which results in clonal exhaustion and diminished numbers of immune cells [2]. Immune activation by both helminths and HIV result in both accelerated CD4+ cells depletion and HIV replication. In that way, infected, activated $CD4^+$ T cells can therefore be prone to depletion by the viral infection/replication cycle and thus increases susceptibility to HIV and other infections.

1.5.3.3. Uncontrolled HIV infection

The increased regulatory cells dampen immune responses not only to parasite-specific antigens but also to bystander antigens, as well as the ability of helminth infections to diverge immune responses [19] result in a high degree of reduced capacity to respond to antigen and immune stimulation. The chronic immune activation is associated with increased apoptosis and cell turnover results in clonal exhaustion and diminished numbers of immune cells, generally reducing the ability of the immune cells to control infectious pathogens including HIV.

One of the consequences of the induction of alternatively activated macrophages by helminths is the conversion of arginine to ornithine. Arginine is required for the production of nitrogen and oxygen intermediate radicals for intracellular killing [19]. Reduction of the innate intracellular killing capability of the immune system promotes uncontrolled intracellular virus propagation.

1.6. Clinical course of *M.tb* infection during helminthiasis and *Mycobacterium tuberculosis* coinfection

1.6.1. Clinical course of M.tb infection

While most individuals who acquire TB infection are able to contain the infection as latent TB infection (LTBI), in a small subset of individuals (5–10%), LTBI may progress to active TB disease, a situation that may be prompted by many factors, among them a weakened immune system. LTBI is often detected by the extent of the immune response to *M.tb* antigens such as purified protein derivative (PPD) or tuberculin skin test (TST). This often measures the release of IFN-γ a hallmark cytokine which is central in the TB immune response [39, 40]. Individuals with LTBI have no clinical or radiological evidence of disease and may live for years without realizing it.

The host mechanisms by which some individuals remain protected while others later develop TB disease remains incompletely understood [41]. However, among the various factors genetic factors of both the host and the pathogen may play an important role in the progression of latent infection to active disease. Other factors such as immune status and the general health condition of the host may also play an important part in this reactivation of latent TB infection. There is now an increasing body of knowledge in the understanding of LTBI being a spectrum of both immunological and microbiological changes rather than binary classification of latent infection and active TB disease [42].

1.6.2. Immune responses to M.tb infection

In pulmonary tuberculosis, generally, the immune response is characterized by the involvement of many different cell types with a predominance of CD4+ T cells [43]. Once the bacilli reach the lower respiratory tract, alveolar macrophages and lung epithelial cells are the first cells that encounter *M.tb* during primary infection. The defense mechanisms by the macrophages include growth inhibition, innate killing mechanism, phagosome-lysosome fusion, generation of reactive oxygen intermediates, and generation of reactive nitrogen intermediates, particularly nitric oxide as well as participation in the adaptive immune response through antigen presentation to T cells [39]. The macrophages also acquire the ability to stimulate type 1 $CD4^+$ Th1 cells or secrete proinflammatory cytokines.

The induction of these inflammatory responses initiates the development of a granuloma [39, 40], where different T-cell populations participate in protective immune responses. Also of note is the effector function of $CD4^+$ Th1 cells which is mainly mediated by the production of cytokines, such as IL-12, TNF-α, and IFN-γ [44, 45]. IFN-γ, which is secreted by activated T cells is an important mediator of the immune response to *M.tb*, as it upregulates antimycobacterial processes and antigen presentation by macrophages [39, 43]. The cytokine IFN-γ and natural killer (NK) cells act as the principal activating factors in the control of mycobacterial infection. The induction of IFN-γ is regulated by IL-12. That the Th1 immune response is critical is highlighted by the increased susceptibility to TB disease in patients treated by TNF-α suppressing drugs such as steroids [41]. The induction of significant Th1 (IL-12, IFN-γ, and TNF-α) and Th17 responses (IL-17 and IL-23) is thus central to the control of tuberculosis [46]. In recent years, the realization that Th17 cells also play a critical role in host's control of TB has come under the spotlight. Studies from animal models have shown that the secretion of IL-17 homologs coupled by IL-22 helps to establish an optimal Th1 response [47].

In sub-Saharan Africa, the immunology of TB is further complicated by the widespread association of TB with HIV, the protracted period of chemotherapy which inadvertently may result in poor treatment compliance and, consequently, the emergence of drug-resistant and multidrug-resistant *M.tb* strains [14]. While there is a licensed vaccine against tuberculosis (BCG) [44, 48], the efficacy of protection it offers against pulmonary tuberculosis is variable and has been shown to wane over time, possibly due to immune alteration by prevalent chronic infections and consequent impairment of immune response to recall antigens [45]. Furthermore, the lack of a point of care diagnostic tool means that TB diagnosis [15] and, consequently, treatment and interruption of transmission does not happen as promptly as required in order to bring the global TB epidemic under control [49].

1.6.3. Mechanisms of interactions between helminths and M.tb

The fact that both *M.tb* and helminth infection are widely distributed geographically, on a global scale, allows for considerable overlap of the infections. By nature helminth infections are chronic and their persistent presence can lead to considerable morbidity [46]. The presence of chronic helminth infection has been known to induce a wide range of immunomodulation mechanisms mainly dominated by a Th2 type immune response and the subsequent release of Th2-related cytokines, such as IL-4, IL-5, and IL-13. On the other hand, the immune responses induced by helminth infection tend to be antagonistic to those induced *by M.tb* infection [45, 50]. While helminth and *M.tb* infection mechanisms are vastly different with *M.tb* being a single-celled organism and helminths being multicellular, several authors have demonstrated the negative association between helminth and mycobacterial infections [51]. The predominant Th2 biased response in helminths has been demonstrated to downregulate the Th1 response that is characteristic and constitutes an essential defense for control of *M.tb*. It has been hypothesized that by creating an antiinflammatory environment, helminths exacerbate *M.tb* infection by antagonizing the protective inflammatory responses needed for the tuberculosis infection.

In addition, helminths can modulate the host's adaptive immune responses by inducing T-regulatory (Treg) cells or secreting antiinflammatory and regulatory cytokines [19, 52]. Such effects could induce a significant inhibitory effect on protective *M.tb*-induced immune responses and/or control of mycobacterial infection. Studies examining association between helminth infection immune response indicators and TB infection have illustrated that worms may impair immunity against mycobacterial infections. Other literature also shows that helminth-infected individuals exhibit markedly lower Th1 type responses and IFN-γ production to *M.tb* antigens relative to dewormed controls [53].

Other studies have further dissected the immune mechanisms triggered by each pathogen in isolation and also investigated their interaction. In this regard, it has been demonstrated that coincident infections with helminths can modulate the strong *M.tb*-specific Th1 immune responses by driving Th2 and/or Treg cells [54]. Furthermore, enhanced Treg function associated with helminth infections have been found to potentially suppress Th1 responses [55] suggesting that intestinal helminth coinfection is associated with a reduced Th1 type immune response in active TB cases while both Th1 and Th17 responses have been shown to be diminished in latent tuberculosis [56].

Many soil-transmitted helminths larvae migrate through the lungs where they can potentially cause an eosinophilic pneumonitis [1]. Eosinophils are induced by a Th2response and may have a deleterious, direct impact on coexisting *M.tb* lung infection which requires a Th1 response. In addition, individuals coinfected with helminths and *M.tb* were also shown to have more advanced disease shown by the number of diseased zones [56]. It is not known whether the helminths could have exacerbated the lung pathology directly or indirectly through an inflammatory process.

Another deleterious interaction between helminths and *M.tb* is the induction of alternatively activated macrophages by helminths [19]. The resultant attenuation of nitric oxide production by these cells inhibits one of the key intracellular killing mechanisms against *M.tb* which can exacerbate the intracellular survival and multiplication of the bacilli. IL-4 stimulates the production of IgE antibodies, classically induced by helminths. High IgE levels have been shown to be inversely associated with a positive tuberculin skin test in Ascaris-infected individuals [57] suggestive of an impaired *M.tb* response associated with helminthiasis.

While a number of studies point to negative impact of helminth infection to the immune responses to mycobacterial infection, other clinical studies also appear to show that helminth infections have little effect on the pathogenesis or pathology of active TB [50]. However, it is important to note that most of these findings are from observational studies with very few longitudinal studies having been performed to examine these hypotheses. In the absence of such long-term longitudinal studies and clinical trials, it remains important to synthesize the current knowledge and present a summary of the findings to date in order to inform policy and further research efforts.

Table 2 summarizes the main mechanisms through which helminth infections are proposed to modulate the HIV and mycobacterium tuberculosis immune responses and course of the diseases.

Effects of helminth infection	Impact on HIV [1]	Impact on Tuberculosis [1, 13]
Cellular alterations		
• **Lower CD4 and higher CD8** • **Alternatively activated macrophages** • **Classic Eosinophilia**	• CD4 T helper cell critical for HIV control: Uncontrolled HIV replication. • Impaired IL-12 production: impaired NK cell intracellular killing of HIV. • Activated eosinophils express CD4 and are infectable by HIV: Increased HIV replication; promotes hetero-and homo-sexual transmission in genital and rectal mucosa.	• CD4 T-cell help essential for protective interferon gamma production: Enhanced TB infection. • Compromised lung anti-tuberculosis defenses. • Reduced NO and RO intracellular killing • Eosinophilia associated with a Th2 response which dampens Th1 anti-tuberculosis responses
Predominant type 2 response Hyper IgE immunoglobulinaemia	• Decreased type 1 CTL responses essential for HIV control: • Uncontrolled HIV replication • Increased HIV replication and apoptosis	• Reduced Th_1 immunity to mycobacteria. Th1 cytokines (TNFα, IL-6 and IL-8) essential for granuloma formation) • Inhibited TLR-mediated protective immunity to TB • Impaired BCG vaccine efficacy.

Effects of helminth infection	Impact on HIV [1]	Impact on Tuberculosis [1, 13]
		• High IgE associated with high TB incidence
Chronic immune activation	• Increased receptor molecules (CD4, CCR5, CXCR4), enhanced HIV entry to cells, cell-cell transmission; Increased transcription factors and virus replication; increased virus transmission in the population.	• Inability to cope with TB, enhanced active pulmonary TB
Regulatory cytokines; specific and generalized immune suppression	• Attenuated immunity increases susceptibility to HIV and faster progression to AIDS.	• Impaired protective TB immunity, • Reactivation of latent TB.
Increased apoptosis	• Increased CD4 T-cell loss, Uncontrolled virus replication	• CD4 T-cell help required for granuloma formation: Inability to contain TB; disseminated infection.

Table 2. Summary key immune interactions between helminthiasis, HIV, and *M.tb* infections.

2. Systematic review of immune interactions during helminth and HIV or *Mycobacterium tuberculosis* coinfection

2.1. Methodology

2.1.1. Search strategy

The electronic database PubMed was searched for relevant articles with no language and time restrictions. Search terms used included a varied combination of "Helminth coinfection and immunity and TB coinfection or TB immunity and HIV coinfection or HIV immunity and Africa." Names of individual species were also permutated in the search terms. Reviews and bibliographies of selected articles were screened to identify additional relevant articles or studies.

2.1.2. Study selection

All retrieved articles were sequentially searched for relevance by title, abstract, and full text. Two authors independently searched through the titles and abstracts to identify potentially relevant papers for inclusion, and consensus on potential eligibility reached with differences resolved through discussion. Full text articles of potentially relevant articles were screened for relevance (**Figure 1**). Articles were excluded from the review if they were (1) not from Africa, (2) based on experimental animal models, (3) review articles, and (4) epidemiological surveys of coinfections without any immunological outcome assessment being reported. The majority of other potentially relevant articles were from countries from Southeast Asia especially India and were therefore excluded.

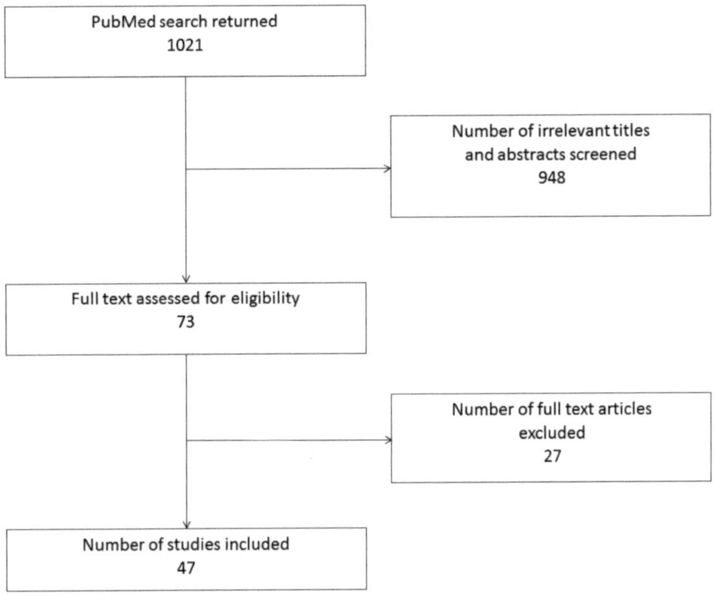

Figure 1. Flow chart showing study selection.

2.1.3. Inclusion criteria for immune interaction

Included were those studies that investigated immune interactions that will worsen HIV disease progression defined by lowered CD4 counts, immunologic failure, increased viral load, impaired immune response, altered immune response-impaired Th1 responses (low IFNg, IL-12); alternatively activated Mø; highly activated immune system; altered distribution of immune cells; altered cytokine profile (Th2 biased; increased Tregs); and anergy (decreased capacity to respond to antigens). For TB, immune interactions were defined by outcomes that result in impaired granuloma formation; impaired Th1 responses (low IFNg, TNFa, IL-12); alternatively activated Mø; altered cytokine profile (Th2 biased; increased Tregs); and anergy (decreased capacity to respond to antigens).

2.1.4. Data extraction

A structured data extraction form was used with the following information being extracted: author(s), year of publication, country, subregion, study design, type of coinfection, study population, and main immunological outcome. Diagnosed and/or reported helminth species were also recorded where available.

3. Results

Literature search in the electronic bibliographic database resulted in 953 unique references and 68 more were extracted from the additional manual searches (**Figure 1**). Of these, 73 articles were considered relevant and assessed for eligibility. A total of 47 relevant articles were identified through PubMed search and cross-referencing of selected articles. Of these 12 were from Southern Africa, 32 from East Africa, and three from West Africa.

A total of 31 relevant studies were on helminth coinfection with HIV, and 18 were from East Africa (seven Ethiopian, five Kenyan, three Ugandan, and four Tanzanian), 10 from Southern Africa (four South African, two Zimbabwean, two Malawian, and one Zambian), and two from West Africa (both from Uganda). In addition, 16 relevant studies were on helminth coinfection with TB, and 13 were from East Africa (nine Ethiopian, three Ugandan, and one Kenyan), two from Southern Africa (all South African), and one from West Africa (Cameroon).

3.1. Helminth and HIV coinfection immunological outcomes

Of the 31 helminth and HIV coinfection studies, 22 (71%) reported some negative effect of helminthiasis on HIV parameters (**Table 3**). Fifteen studies investigated the effects of treating helminth infection on HIV viral load, CD4 count, immune activation, or disease progression. Eight of the 15 (53%) reported a positive impact of treating worm infection by either stabilizing or decreasing viral load [59, 62, 65, 73] or increasing or stabilizing CD4+ counts [16, 62, 65, 68, 82] or decreasing IgE levels [85] and seven reported no impact of deworming [16, 34, 63, 64, 72, 77, 80], two of which reported no benefit of empiric deworming of HIV- and helminth-coinfected individuals [73, 79]. Two studies reported high immune activation associated with coinfection [71, 80] which was not affected by anthelminthic treatment [80]. Five studies reported increased HIV coreceptor molecules CCR5, CXCR4 [16, 22, 60, 71, 81], or CD4 molecules [70], among helminth-infected individuals. One study reported increased odds of antiretroviral treatment immunological failure induced by helminthiasis [74], while another reported increased expression of inflammatory markers [66] and another showed increased HIV susceptibility of peripheral blood monocytes obtained from helminth-infected individuals [58]. An increased risk of mother-to-child transmission by helminth-infected mothers was reported in one study [61]. One study reported decreased capacity to proliferate in response to antigen stimulation and reduced type I cytokines among HIV-/helminth-infected individuals [78].

Authors	Year	Country	Subregion	Study design	Sample size	Coinfections and study population	Immunological outcomes
Shapira-Nahor et al. [58]	1998	Ethiopia	East Africa			PBMCs of helminth-infected, immune-activated individuals	Increased HIV susceptibility of PBMCs from helminth-infected individuals.
Lawn et al. [34]	2000	Kenya	East Africa	Prospective cohort	30	Schistosomiasis HIV-infected persons	No correlation between eradication of Schistosoma infection and reduction in HIV load. Instead, a

Authors	Year	Country	Subregion	Study design	Sample size	Coinfections and study population	Immunological outcomes
							transient posttreatment interval-dependent increase in viral load was found.
Wolday et al. [59]	2002	Ethiopia	East Africa	Prospective cohort	56	Helminth-infected and noninfected in asymptomatic HIV-1-infected individuals	At baseline heavier egg load was associated with higher virus load. At 6 months' follow-up, there was a mean decrease of −0.36 log10 in HIV load among 13 successfully treated participants.
Elliot et al. [60]	2003	Uganda	East Africa	Prospective	68	Helminth-infected and uninfected HIV-1 positive, ART-naive individuals	There was increased expression of HIV coreceptor molecules CCR5 and CXCR4 on cells of *Schistosoma*-infected adults.
Secor et al. [22]	2003	Kenya	East Africa	Prospective		*Schistosoma*-infected HIV-1-positive and negative individuals	Increased expression of HIV coreceptor molecules CCR5 and CXCR4 on cells of *Schistosoma*-infected adults.
Gallagher et al. [61]	2005	Kenya	East Africa	Retrospective cohort	936	Helminth and/or malaria-infected HIV-positive and HIV-negative pregnant women	Helminth-infected mothers had in increased risk for MTCT of HIV compared to uninfected mothers, which correlated with cord blood lymphocytes production of interleukin-5/ interleukin-13 in response to helminth antigens.
Kallestrup et al. [62]	2005	Zimbabwe	Southern Africa	Prospective cohort	287	Schistosomiasis in individuals with or without HIV-1 infection	Early treatment of schistosomiasis was associated with a significant increase in CD4 counts, and

Authors	Year	Country	Subregion	Study design	Sample size	Coinfections and study population	Immunological outcomes
							arrested increase in viral load, while there was an increase in HIV RNA load in the delayed-treatment group.
Modjarrad et al. [63]	2005	Zambia	Southern Africa	Prospective	428	Helminth-infected and uninfected HIV-1 asymptomatic individuals	No significant association between treatment of helminths and reduction of viral load was found
Hosseinipour et al. [64]	2007	Malawi	Southern Africa	Prospective	389	Helminths in HIV-uninfected and HIV-infected individuals	Neither helminth parasitic infection nor treatment thereof had an impact on HIV viral load.
Nielsen et al. [65]	2007	Tanzania	East Africa	RCT	27	Filarial parasite-infected and uninfected HIV-infected individuals	A significant decrease in HIV load (54%) and an insignificant increase in CD4% were observed in the HIV-positive individuals with filarial co-infection at 12 weeks after treatment.
Zinyama-Gutsire et al. [66]	2009	Zimbabwe	Southern Africa	Prospective cohort	379	Schistosomiasis infection and HIV-1 co-infection	*S. haematobium*- and *S. mansoni*-infected participants had significantly higher MBL levels than uninfected partcipants. All MBL2 variants were not associated with HIV-1 infection but promoter variants LY and LL were significantly associated with *S. haematobium* infection.
Babatunde et al. [67]	2010	Nigeria	Western Africa	Cross-sectional	135	Intestinal parasites in HIV patients	Patients with CD4+ count <200/μl had more coccidian parasites in their

Authors	Year	Country	Subregion	Study design	Sample size	Coinfections and study population	Immunological outcomes
							stool and also had higher prevalence of intestinal polyparasitism ranging from 2 to 4 different species per stool sample.
Walson et al. [68]	2010	Kenya	East Africa	RTC	1551	Helminth co-infection in HIV-1-infected adults	Treatment of A. lumbricoides with albendazole in HIV-1coinfected adults resulted in significantly increased CD4 cell counts during 3-month follow-up.
Akinbo et al. [69]	2011	Nigeria	West Africa	Serial sampling method	2000	Intestinal parasites in HIV-infected patients	Anaemia was associated with CD4 count while Cryptosporidium species, Ascaris lumbricoides, hookworm, and Taenia species were the intestinal parasitic agents associated with anemia.
Jourdan et al. [70]	2011	Malawi	Southern Africa		89	Women with S. haematobium	S. haematobium may significantly increase the density of HIV target cells (CD4+ T lymphocytes and macrophages) in the female genitals, creating a beneficial setting for HIV transmission
Mkhize-Kwitshana et al. [71]	2011	South Africa	Southern Africa	Cross-sectional	62	Helminth and HIV singly infected, dual-infected and uninfected individuals	People with both helminth egg excretion and high Ascaris-IgE levels had dysregulated immune cells, eosinophilia, higher viral loads with more immune activation (HLADR, CCR-5 and

Authors	Year	Country	Subregion	Study design	Sample size	Coinfections and study population	Immunological outcomes
							CD38 upregulated). A modified Th2 helminth response in individuals with egg positive stools and low Ascaris IgE showed a better HIV related immune profile.
Idindili [72]	2012	Tanzania	Eastern Africa	Longitudinal descriptive	421	Parasitic infections in HIV-infected patients	Patients coinfected with helminths and HIV had higher HIV p24, and parasite-infected patients had lower CD4 cell counts than parasite free patients, but this was not statistically significant. Multiple infection was associated with CD4+ T cells <200/μl compared to one parasite coinfection.
Walson et al. [73]	2012	Kenya	East Africa	RCT	948	Helminth and helminth-coinfected adults	There was no evidence of the effect of empiric deworming in the delaying of HIV disease progression in adults with HIV
Webb et al. [74]	2012	Uganda	East Africa	RCT	264	Helminths in HIV-infected pregnant women	Hookworm and Trichuris infections were associated with higher mean viral load at enrolment, and there $p = 0.05$ was some evidence that albendazole reduced viral load at 6 weeks posttreatment ($p = 0.05$).
Efraim et al. [75]	2013	Tanzania	East Africa	Retrospective cohort study	351	Schistosome infection in HIV-infected patients' responses on ART	Odds of developing immunological failure were four times greater in patients with

Authors	Year	Country	Subregion	Study design	Sample size	Coinfections and study population	Immunological outcomes
							schistosome coinfection. Schistosome-infected patients also had significantly lower CD4 count increases on ART than schistosome-uninfected patients.
Mulu et al. [76]	2013	Ethiopia	Eastern Africa		220	Helminthic-infected and uninfected HIV-1 patients	Twelve weeks after antihelminthic treatment, helminth infestations and their treatment had no significant effect on CD4+ T-cell counts. However, helminth-infested individuals had a higher level of CD8 (+) T cells at baseline, which was significantly reduced at 12 weeks after antihelminthic treatment.
Gebreegziabiher et al. [77]	2014	Ethopia	East Africa	Cross-sectional	85	Helminth-HIV-co-infected pregnant women	There was no significant difference in IL-4 response of CBMCs between helminth negative and positive participants. Maternal helminth infection had a significant association with the IFN-γ response of CBMCs, total IgE, and cross-placental transfer of TB-specific IgG.
Mkhize-Kwitshana et al. [78]	2014	South Africa	Southern Africa	Cross-sectional	62	Helminth and HIV singly infected, dually infected and uninfected individuals	Dual HIV/helminth infection with egg excretion and/or high Ascaris IgE phenotype may be linked with poor proliferative capacity

Authors	Year	Country	Subregion	Study design	Sample size	Coinfections and study population	Immunological outcomes
							and deleterious cytokine profile with regards to HIV control.
Lankowski et al. [79]	2014	Uganda	East Africa	Retrospective observational	5379	Helminth in HIV-infected adults on ART	Empiric deworming of HIV-infected individuals on ART conferred no significant generalized benefit on subsequent CD4 count recovery. A significant association was observed exclusively in females and during the initial year on ART
Chachage et al. [80]	2014	Tanzania	Eastern Africa	Prospective cohort	386	Helminth coinfection with HIV in adults	Trichuris, Ascaris, and *S. mansoni* infections correlate with increased expression of T-cell activation markers with relatively little effect of helminth treatment compared to helminth-negative controls. Contrary, hookworm infection was associated with slightly decreased frequency of HLA-DR expressing.
Kleppa et al. [16]	2014	South Africa	Southern Africa	Prospective cohort	853	Female genital schistosomiasis and HIV target cell density and expression of the HIV co-receptor CCR5 in blood and cervical cytobrush samples	Increased expression of CD14+ monocytes and CCR4+ CD4 cells among schstosomiasis-infected (FGS +)individuals (FGS+) than from FGS- women (4.7% vs. 1.5%, p=0.018) in blood and genital samples which decreased significantly in both

Authors	Year	Country	Subregion	Study design	Sample size	Coinfections and study population	Immunological outcomes
							compartments after anti-schistosomal treatment (p= 0.043).
Noormahomed et al. [81]	2014	Mozambique	Southern Africa	Cross-sectional	601	Cysticercosis, Schistosomiasis, Toxocariasis, and Echinococcosis in HIV patients	Patients with CD4+ count between 200 and 500/μl had a higher seroprevalence to all helminths than those with less than 200/μl cells and those with more than 500 cells/μl.
Abossie and Petros [82]	2015	Ethiopia	East Africa		97	Helminth/HIV coinfection	CD4+ T-cell count in the *Ascaris lumbricoides*/HIV-coinfected was significantly higher and after 15 weeks and 6 months postantihelminthics treatment, respectively. Also, after antihelminthic therapy, the CD4+ T-cell count significantly increased in all treated helminth infections.
Kleppa et al. [83]	2015	South Africa	Southern Africa	Cross-sectional	792	S. haematobium infection and in HIV infected	Urogenital schistosomiasis does not influence the number of circulating CD4 cells.
Mengist et al. [84]	2015	Ethiopia	East Africa	Cross-sectional	550	Intestinal parasitosis in HAART initiated and HAART naive pediatric HIV patients	Hook worm and Taenia species were IPs associated with CD4+ T-cell counts <350 cells/μl in HAART naive patients
Mulu et a [85]	2015	Ethiopia	East Africa	Prospective cohort	130	Helminth-infected and uninfected HIV-infected individuals	Helminths showed a high level of serum IgE compared to HIV patients without helminths

Authors	Year	Country	Subregion	Study design	Sample size	Coinfections and study population	Immunological outcomes
							coinfection. A significant decline in serum IgE level was observed 12 weeks after deworming and ART of symptomatic HIV-infected patients with and helminths coinfection. There was no significant decrease in serum IgE level among asymptomatic HIV-infected individuals.

Table 3. Helminth HIV coinfection studies included in the systematic literature review.

As indicated in the summary results, the overall picture indicates that while some studies reported no impact (on HIV infection) of deworming on helminth-infected individuals, the majority actually showed a beneficial effect. Other studies that analyzed different aspects such as immune activation, proliferative capacity, inflammatory markers, and expression of coreceptor molecules indicated a negative impact of helminth infection on HIV disease markers. Indeed a sizeable proportion of these also failed to show any negative interaction between helminths and HIV.

3.2. Helminth TB coinfection immunological outcome

The 16 helminth and TB coinfection studies investigated (1) the general immune responses of helminthiasis with mycobacterial coinfections and (2) effect of intestinal helminths on the immune response to naturally immunized or BCG-vaccinated humans, and (3) effect of antituberculosis chemotherapy on helminth-infected TB patients with and without HIV (**Table 4**). Generally, immune response studies of helminth- and mycobacterial-coinfected individuals revealed that co-infection with helminths appear to dampen the proinflammatory cytokine response while promoting a regulatory/Th2-mediated immune response [90]. Studies that analyzed the interaction of helminth infection and response to *M.tb* antigen, purified protein derivative (PPD), also showed a T-cell-mediated immune response skewed toward a Th2 type response against helminth and PPD antigens. Similarly, BCG-vaccinated individuals infected with various helminths species also exhibited attenuated T-cell and skin responses with Malhotra et al. reporting a 26-fold magnitude difference in IFN-gamma production in BCG-vaccinated infants who were not exposed versus those who were prenatally exposed to filariae and schistosomes [96, 93]. Thus, chronic worm infection was noted to reduce the immunogenicity of BCG in humans [86]. In their study, Adams et al. reported that TB patients were observed to have a higher total IgE and Ascaris-specific IgE (in comparison to controls), which declined significantly after treatment [87]. IgE levels were reported to be significantly higher in TB patients coinfected with HIV and helminths compared to those without helminth coinfection with anti-TB chemotherapy significantly reducing the serum IgE levels in HIV seronegative TB patients. Several other studies also showed that the immune response in helminth-TB-coinfected individuals was characterized by elevated IgE levels [87, 91]. Elliott et al. also reported a significant association between eosinophilia, elevated IgE levels, and asymptomatic infection which improved with anti-TB treatment [89]. Asymptomatic helminth infection was also observed to be associated with increased regulatory T-cell and Th2 type immune responses by the same authors [92].

Authors	Year	Country	Subregion	Study design	Sample size	Coinfections and study population	Immunological outcome
Malhotra et al. [86]	1999	Kenya	East Africa	Cross-sectional	33	Schistosoma filariasis-infected mothers and BCG-vaccinated infants and 2–10 year-olds	T-cell IFN-γ production evaluated 10–14 months after BCG vaccination was 26-fold higher for infants who were not sensitized to filariae or schistosomes *in utero* relative to subjects who experienced prenatal sensitization.
Adams et al. [87]	1999	South Africa	Southern Africa		740		TB patients had higher total IgE and Ascaris-specific IgE than controls before TB treatment and declined after treatment. Tuberculin induration correlated inversely with IgE in patients but not in controls.
Stewart et al. [88]	1999	Cameroon	West Africa		50	Helminth and mycobacterial infections in 5–16 year olds	There was a MF density-related downregulation of cellular responsiveness and age-related skewing toward type 2 which was paralleled in response to both the helminth antigen and PPD.
Elias et al. [53]	2001	Ethiopia	East Africa	Prospective cohort	240	Intestinal helminths in naturally immunized or BCG-vaccinated College students	BCG-vaccinated individuals infected with various helminths had attenuated T-cell and skin test responses.
Eliot et al. [89]	2003	Uganda	East Africa	Prospective follow-up	625	Helminth and TB in adult	High rates of subsequent progression to active TB were associated with eosinophil counts ⊚ 0.4 × 109/L at enrolment. (Eosinophilia associated

Authors	Year	Country	Subregion	Study design	Sample size	Coinfections and study population	Immunological outcome
							with schstosomiasis in this study).
Kassu et al. [90]	2003	Ethiopia	East Africa	Long-term cohort	64	Parasitic infection in HIV-1-infected and uninfected adult	Incidental intestinal parasitic infections resulted in a significant increase in memory CD4+ T-cell numbers both in HIV-negative and HIV-positive subjects. There was also a significant increase in the percentage of CD8+ HLA-DR+ T cells ($p < 0.05$) in HIV-positive subjects coinfected with parasites.
Kassu et al. [91]	2004	Ethiopia	East Africa	Consecutive sampling	241	Tuberculosis patients with or without intestinal helminthic infection and/or HIV infection	IgE level was significantly higher in patients coinfected with intestinal helminthes and HIV compared to those infected with helminthes or without coinfection. Antituberculosis chemotherapy significantly reduced serum IgE levels in HIV seronegative tuberculosis patients.
Elias et al. [92]	2006	Ethiopia	East Africa	Case control	Cases (n = 230) Control (n = 510)	Helminth infections in active tuberculosis patients	The odds of being a TB patient increased with the number of helminth species per person: in individuals with monoinfection it was 4.3 (95% CI 2.8–6.8); in people infected with two species was 4.7 (95% CI 2.5–8.7), and in patients infected with three or more helminths was 12.2 (3.9–52.6).
Elias et al. [93]	2008	Ethiopia	East Africa		280	Volunteers with prior mycobacterial infection and asymptomatic helminths infection	Chronic worm infection reduces the immunogenicity of BCG in humans and this was associated with increased TGF-beta production but not with enhanced Th2 immune response.
Webb et al. [94]	2011	Uganda	East Africa	RCT	Women (n =	Helminth- and HIV-infected women and	Neither albendazole nor praziquantel treatments

Authors	Year	Country	Subregion	Study design	Sample size	Coinfections and study population	Immunological outcome
					2356) Infants (n = 1115)	BCG-vaccinated infants	affected infant response to BCG, tetanus, or measles immunization.
Abate et al. [94]	2012	Ethiopia	East Africa	Consecutive sampling	295	Helminth=infected TB patients with and without HIV	Eosinophilia and elevated IgE levels were significantly associated with asymptomatic helminth infection. During TB treatment, the worm infection rate of HIV+/TB patients declined from 31% (10/32) at week 0 to 9% (3/32) at week 2 of TB treatment, whereas HIV −/TB patients showed no change from baseline to week 2, 29% (13/45) vs. 22.2% (10/45).
van Soelen et al. [57]	2012	South Africa	Southern Africa	Cross-sectional	271	A. lumbricoides and *M.tb* in children	There was an inverse association between Ascaris IgE status and a positive TST (OR = 0.6, p = 0.08), when adjusted for age, and *M.tb* contact score. The effect of being Ascaris IgE positive significantly reduced the odds of being TST positive amongst younger children while this effect weakened with increasing age.
Wassie et al. [95]	2013	Ethiopia	East Africa	Cross-sectional	245	Healthy school children aged from 12 to 20 years	A subset of children who had a positive QuantIFERON™ result but a negative tuberculin skin test.
Biraro et al. [96]	2014	Uganda	East Africa	Prospective cohort	291?	Helminth-coinfected and newly infected TB patients	Household contacts with LTBI had elevated cytokine responses to tuberculosis antigens but coinfections had little effect on cytokine responses.
Gebreegziabihe et al. [77]	2014	Ethiopia	East Africa	Cross-sectional	85	Helminth infections in pregnant women and immunity after infection with TB and neonatal	The IFN-γ response of CBMCs to ESAT-6/CFP-10 cocktail was significantly lower in helminth-positive than helminth-negative

Authors	Year	Country	Subregion	Study design	Sample size	Coinfections and study population	Immunological outcome
						immune function and immunity to TB	participants. Maternal helminth infection had a significant negative association with the IFN-γ response of CBMCs, total IgE, and cross placental transfer of TB specific IgG.
Abate et al. [97]	2015	Ethiopia	East Africa	Consecutive sampling	121	Helminth-infected TB patients	Asymptomatic helminth infection is associated with increased regulatory T-cell and Th2- type responses and a lower rate of sputum smear positivity

Table 4. Helminth TB coinfection studies included in the systematic literature review.

A clinical trial by Webb et al. reported that neither treatment with albendazole nor praziquatel affected infant BCG immune responses [94]. Another interesting finding was the increased odds of being a TB patient for individuals who had more than one species of helminths reported by Elias et al. [92]. In newly infected/latently infected TB household contacts, cytokine responses to TB antigens were higher compared to coinfected individuals [96]. Furthermore, several studies showed that chronic worm infection reduces the immunogenicity of BCG in humans [96, 98]. Improved mycobacterial antigen-specific cellular responses in BCG-vaccinated persons were observed after treatment of helminthes.

4. Discussion

The extent of convergent distribution of tuberculosis, HIV, and helminth infection in sub-Saharan Africa is evident in the selected literature in this review. Likewise, the contrasting immune responses elicited by the extracellular helminthic parasites and intracellular HIV and *M.tb* infections provide an immunobiologically plausible support for the antagonistic interaction in coinfected hosts The review extracted 47 studies that investigated the immunological interactions between helminthiasis and HIV and/or mycobacterium tuberculosis. The studies were spread across the Western, Southern, and East Africa, the latter having the most relevant articles (31 of 46) and the Western Africa the least (three articles). The scarcity of such studies in West Africa may be due to that fact that this region, together with East Africa, has the lowest HIV/AIDS burden compared to the worst affected Southern region. Interestingly though, the East African region has a leading number of such investigations.

4.1. Immune response to helminths and HIV coinfection

Immunological consequences of coinfection with HIV and helminth infections were also investigated. Different aspects of immunological outcomes were measured, and some studies did not find evidence of a negative interaction, others indicated a deleterious effect of helminthiasis. The hallmark of helminth infections—(i) cellular changes, (ii) immune activation, (iii) a Th2 biased immune profile, and (iv) increased regulatory cells associated with anergy were addressed by the studies reviewed as well as other immune-related aspects of HIV such as viral replication, increased susceptibility to HIV, and increased risk of transmission. Cellular changes induced by helminthiasis include reduction of the central adaptive immune response subset—the CD4+ cells. Helminth infections have been shown to be associated with decreased frequencies of these cells [21].

It is generally accepted that a CD4 count less than 200 cells/μl predisposes HIV-infected persons to opportunistic infections. Several investigations in this review demonstrated an association between reduction of these cells and helminthiasis [67, 81, 84]. In their study, Akinbo et al. [69] showed that a CD4 count of less than 200 cells/μl resulted in a significantly higher prevalence of intestinal parasitic infections and Idindili et al. [72] reported that multiple infection was associated with CD4+ T cells <200/μl compared to one parasite coinfection. In addition, the prevalence of anemia in HIV-infected patients is high, while low CD4 count is a significant risk factor of acquiring anemia. Some parasite species also induce anemia, such as the Trichuris which burrow and suck blood from the small intestine of infected individuals. Akinbo et al. [69] further demonstrated that *A. lumbricoides*, hookworm, and Taenia species in HIV-infected individuals are parasitic agents associated with anemia. These human studies lend support to the negative association between immune modulation by helminthiasis and HIV infection. However, one study in this review failed to show this association, where urogenital schistosomiasis was not found to influence the number of circulating CD4+ cells [83].

Another change in the distribution of peripheral blood cells during helminthiasis is marked increase in eosinophils, the key effector cells which play a specialized role in immunity to helminths. These cells together with IgE are produced by CD4+ Th2 cells, indicating a predominance of these cells during helminthiasis. In the current review, the significant decline of serum IgE level 12 weeks after deworming of both symptomatic and asymptomatic patients [85] confirms the Th2 immune response induced by helminths [66]. As indicated earlier, increased numbers of activated eosinophils that express CD4 molecules provide an extra supply of HIV target cells at convenient sites for HIV infection during sexual encounter in homosexual (rectal) or heterosexual (genital) mucosa of helminth-infected sexual partners. Furthermore, the helminth-induced Th2 polarized immune response spills over to bystander cells, influences the response to other nonparasite antigens, and skews them toward a Th2 phenotype [19]. In humans, ascariasis was associated with impaired Th1 responses to vibrio cholera [99], which was later improved by deworming—treatment of Ascaris lumbricoides resulted in enhanced antivibrio antibody production [100]. Likewise, significantly impaired proliferative, T helper 1 (IL-2 and interferon γ) tetanus responses have been documented in tetanus toxoid-vaccinated, onchocerciasis-infected children [101]. Gopinath et al. attributed all these phenomena to a Th2-biased immune profile induced by helminths.

Thirty-two cases of new HIV cases were recorded in a 5-year cohort study involving 1055 individuals who were initially HIV negative, with a confirmed prior filarial infection [102]. This study demonstrated for the first time in humans, a significantly increased risk of HIV acquisition among lymphatic filariasis-infected individuals, lending strong support to the *in vitro* study in this review that showed increased HIV susceptibility of PBMCs obtained from filarial-infected individuals [58]. In another study, PBMCs from filarial-infected individuals were also shown to be more susceptible to HIV infection [103]. In this study, viral replication as measured by reverse transcriptase (RT) values were higher but not statistically significant among the infected compared to the uninfected group and viral replication was significantly reduced 1–2 years after treatment of filariasis. These *in vitro* findings, together with the four studies extracted in the current review that reported increased expression of HIV coreceptors among filarial- or schistosoma-infected individuals [16, 22, 60, 71], provide strong suggestive evidence of increasing susceptibility to HIV by helminthiasis. These exemplify suggestive evidence of a negative immune regulation consequence of helminthiasis on HIV control.

Chronic immune activation resulting from prolonged exposure to helminths is widely described during helminthiasis [2, 19]. In this review two studies reported highly activated immune profiles among HIV- and helminth-coinfected adults [71, 80]. Immune activation was shown to correlate better with HIV disease progression and CD4+ cell decline [30]. Indeed, treatment of parasitic infections showed a tendency to reduce the activation suggesting that, together with other community-based intervention strategies, such treatment could be used to downregulate immune activation and hence protect the host from being easily infected by HIV. In a practical illustration of the deleterious effects of immune activation was the study by Rizardi et al. [104] where simultaneous initiation of antiretroviral therapy (ART) and administration of cyclosporin-A (immunosuppressant) improved CD4 counts restitution in HIV-infected individuals compared to their ART-only counterparts [105]. This finding strongly demonstrated the negative relationship between immune activation and HIV pathogenesis, and implications thereof for helminthiasis-induced chronic immune activation on HIV aggravation.

In this review, helminths have been shown to modulate other aspects of the immune system with potential negative consequences to other microbes. Mannose-binding lectin, part of the innate mechanism required for nonspecific pathogen binding of foreign antigens, was increased among schistosoma-infected individuals [66], which could impair this pathway of immune response for other pathogens. In addition, other deleterious effects of helminthiasis, such as increased risks of mother-to-child transmission of HIV [61] and immunological failure on ART [75], as well as increased levels of HIV p24 (indicative of high virus load) [73], were reported in studies extracted in the review. Decreased proliferative capacity of lymphocytes and reduced type 1 cytokines among HIV-helminth coinfected individuals [78] were also reported.

One of the major attempts at addressing the possible deleterious effect of helminthiasis on HIV infection is to determine whether deworming would reverse the immune dysregulation induced by helminths among HIV-infected individuals. Like in many reported studies, the results remain controversial. Of the 15 such studies, seven reported no impact of deworming coinfected individuals, one even reported a transient increase in viral load after anthelminthic treatment [34]. On the other hand, eight of the 15 studies reported a positive effect of deworming coinfected individuals, some reported an arrest or reduction of viral load after antihelminthic treatment or an increase in CD4+ counts. Kleppa et al. [16] reported a significant reduction of CD4+ CCR5 expressing T cells and monocytes in blood and vaginal samples after antischistosomial treatment among young women. Mulu et al. [85], on the other hand, reported a reduction of IgE levels among helminth-infected individuals after deworming, supporting the concept that deworming positively impacts HIV/AIDS diseases progression.

In one study in Kenya, Walson et al. reported that albendazole-treatment of *Ascaris lumbricoides* resulted in a significant increase in CD4+ counts in HIV-helminth-coinfected adults [68]. Two years later the authors reported no benefit of empiric deworming of HIV coinfected individuals in the same country [73]. Lawonski et al. [79] also reported no general benefit of deworming helminth-HIV-coinfected individuals. Nonetheless, the latest Cochrane review (last updated on the 29 September 2015) which included eight trials that enrolled 1612 participants concluded that there is low quality evidence that treating helminth infections in HIV-infected adults may have small short-term benefits on HIV disease progression and that deworming does not have serious adverse effects [105]. It is important to note that conclusive results of empiric deworming of helminth- and HIV/*M.tb*-coinfected individuals are required. This approach would be more cost-effective compared to targeted deworming of confirmed helminth-infected individuals. The diagnosis and confirmation of helminthiasis is expensive as it requires laboratory equipment such as microscopes, culture systems for some species such as for the strongyloides larva, ELISA readers and washers for serological confirmation in order to increase the low sensitivity of microscopy, as well as a well-trained microscopist. Empiric deworming will obviate the need for such expensive resources, particularly in poorly resourced settings where these three infections frequently coexist.

4.2. Immune response to helminth and TB coinfection

Among 16 studies that analyzed immunological interactions between helminths and *M.tb* coinfection there was evidence for a reduction in type 1 dependent cellular responses as shown by decreased IFNγ production by T cells [77, 86] or low tuberculin skin test responses [57]. A study by Guadalupe et al. [106] showed evidence of increased frequencies of IL-4 and IFNγ CD4+ responses to Ascaris lumbricoides antigen stimulation in the cord blood of neonates born of infected mothers. Frequencies of IFN-γ and IL-4 expressing CD4+ T cells in newborns born of infected mothers were attenuated compared to those of noninfected mothers [106]. The authors assert that the data provide evidence of *in utero* sensitization to Ascaris lumbricoides, and raise the possibility that the immunological effects of infection start in the fetus. In an earlier study, Malhotra et al. also reported related findings where they observed infants who had experienced prenatal sensitization [86]. In such infants, the immune response to BGC vaccination was shown to be biased against the Th1 response in those infants who were exposed to filiarae or schistosomes compared to those who were not exposed and that this immune status persists beyond infancy. These findings indicate a reduction of BCG immunogenicity or impaired TST responses by chronic helminth infection, which were further corroborated by Gebreegziabiher et al. [77]. Thus, helminth infections have significant practical implications and pose a significant threat to the effectiveness of the BCG vaccine, particularly in areas with a high burden of helminth and TB infections.

http://dx.doi.org/10.5772/106429

In another study, evidence of elevated Th2 responses, a classic feature of helminthiasis was reported either through high total and Ascaris-specific IgE which declined after TB treatment [87, 97] or IgE and eosinophilia, the latter associated with high rates of progression to active TB disease [89]. In addition, helminth-induced upregulation of regulatory cells and Th2 responses were also associated with lower rate of sputum positivity [97]. These findings indicate that helminths may have adverse consequences for TB disease and diagnostic efforts, directly impacting on transmission control of TB disease. Yet another study reported increased odds of having TB disease among helminth-infected individuals [92]. However, few studies did not find such an interaction, for example, albendazole treatment did not have any effect on BCG immune response in infants while Biraro and coworkers reported that helminth-latent TB coinfection had no effect on cytokine responses to TB antigens [94, 96]. In one Ethiopian study the immune responses to quantiferon and TST antigens in healthy children from an endemic setting were found to be discordant [95].

In the main, these studies suggest a negative relationship between helminth infection and TB. By and large, most of the studies showed that coinfection with helminth infection dampens the immune response to both latent and active disease. This effect of a suppressed characteristic antitubercular Th 1 immune response was observed regardless of age as the studies reported corroborative findings for prenatally/*in utero* sensitized infants, young children, adolescents, and adults alike. These findings have important implications in the prevention (vaccination) and control of TB in helminth-TB endemic regions such as much of the developing world. With helminthiasis being a silent disease and so very often asymptomatic, the results we present in this study suggest that important policy and public health measures must be adopted in order to bring under control or eliminate the two infections. An important intervention would be comprehensive medical packages for suspected TB-helminth infections particularly in endemic areas. In areas of the world with a high burden of HIV and TB, the WHO policy now recommends screening for HIV for all TB patients and vice versa. In this same way our results suggests that investigating for asymptomatic helminth infections in any suspected TB cases may have important implications for the control of TB in coinfected individuals.

We however note that the results presented here were mainly derived from observational and cross-sectional studies with very few clinical studies. Although a randomized clinical trial could potentially be useful in providing more definitive evidence the ethical and cost implications of conducting such a study are difficult to justify. Prospective studies could also be useful to determine whether the immune system rebounces after the treatment of both TB and helminth infections. Although a few such studies were reported in the studies we examined, the study design and research questions did not clearly address this question, hence the findings were not very definitive.

5. Conclusion

The reviewed studies, like all others in this field have provided results in support and against the hypothesis that chronic infection with helminths result in poor immunological and disease outcomes in coinfected hosts. However, there is evidence of immune alteration such as reduced type 1 responses and increased Th2 and regulatory responses induced by helminth infection in humans. Evidence for possible vaccine inefficiency, increased risks of mother-to-child transmission, and unfavorable treatment outcomes shown in some of these studies confirm the likelihood of a serious public health implication for both major infectious organisms, HIV, and *M.tb*. In the face of the huge financial investments needed for vaccine development, these efforts must be accompanied by insightful consideration of the fact that those vaccines which ultimately reach the market will be rolled out in areas where there is a high likelihood of widespread immune regulation. The fact that TB and helminths are diseases of poverty, contrasts the large financial investment demand for vaccine and drug development with a discouraging likelihood of a low return. Other mechanisms are therefore required to counter widespread immune activation and regulation among the poor individuals exposed to coinfections, as shown in this review. More studies particularly in Southern Africa are needed to increase the much sought evidence of the impact of deworming among HIV-infected individuals as this seems the most feasible, cost-effective intervention with little or no serious adverse effects. Lastly, with expansion of ART and increased access to HIV treatment, the effects of helminths on antiretroviral treatment efficacy also need serious consideration, in light of the suggestive evidence of possible immunologic failure due to helminth coinfection.

Author details

Zilungile L. Mkhize-Kwitshana[1*], Rebecca Tadokera[2] and Musawenkosi H.L. Mabaso[3]

*Address all correspondence to: kwitshanazl@mut.ac.za

1 Mangosuthu University of Technology & University of KwaZulu-Natal, Durban, South Africa

2 HAST, Human Sciences Research Council, Cape Town, South Africa

3 HAST, Human Sciences Research Council, Durban, South Africa

References

[1] Chiodini PL, Moody AH, Manser DW Britton R. The Atlas of Medical Helminthology and Protozoology, 4th ed, 2003. Churchill Livingstone; China. ISBN 0443 06268 4

[2] Borkow G, Bentwich Z. Chronic immune activation associated with chronic helminthic and Human Immunodeficency Virus infections: Role of hyporesponsiveness and anergy. Clinical Microbiology Reviews. 2004; 17(4): 1012–1030.

[3] Global Atlas of Helminth Infections. Available at http://www.thiswormyworld.org/maps/by-region/africa [Accessed 2016-07-28].

[4] Soil Transmitted Helminths WHO Factsheet. Available at http://www.who.int/mediacentre/factsheets/fs366/en/ Updated March 2016. [Accessed: 2016-07-31].

[5] World Health Organization: WHO Technical Series Report, 912. Prevention and control of schistosomiasis and soil-transmitted helminthiasis. 2002. Geneva: World Health Organization.

[6] Pullan RL, Smith JL, Jasrasaria R, Brooker SJ. Global numbers of infection and disease burden of soil transmitted helminth infections in 2010. Parasites & Vectors. 2014; 7: 37. doi: 10.1186/1756-3305-7-37

[7] Bundy D, Sher A, Michael E. Good worms or bad worms: do worm infections affect the epidemiological patterns of other diseases? Parasitology Today. 2000; 16: 273–274.

[8] Castro GA. Helminths: Structure, Classification, Growth, and Development. In: Baron S, editor. Medical Microbiology, 4th ed. Galveston (TX); 1996. Chapter 86.

[9] AIDS by the Numbers. UNAIDS 2016. Available at http://www.unaids.org/en/resources/documents/2016/AIDS-by-the-numbers [Accessed 22016-0901].

[10] WHO HIV Factsheet 2014. Available at http://www.who.int/gho/hiv/en/ [Accessed 2016-09-01].

[11] UNAIDS Global HIV/AIDS statistics. Available at http://www.avert.org/global-hiv-and-aids-statistics[Accessed 2016-09-01].

[12] Glaziou P, Floyd K, Raviglione M. Global burden and epidemiology of tuberculosis. Clinics in Chest Medicine. 2009; 30(4): 621–36–vii.

[13] WHO. Global Tuberculosis Report, 2015. pp. 1–204.

[14] Kasprowicz VO, Achkar JM, Wilson D. The tuberculosis and HIV epidemic in South Africa and the KwaZulu-Natal Research Institute for Tuberculosis and HIV. Journal of Infectious Diseases. 2011; 204 (Suppl 4): S1099–S1101.

[15] Pai M, Schito M. Tuberculosis diagnostics in 2015: landscape, priorities, needs, and prospects. Journal of Infectious Diseases. 2015; 211 (Suppl 2): S21–S28.

[16] Kleppa E, Ramsuran V, Zulu S, Karlsen GH, Bere A, Passmore J-AS, Ndhlovu P, Lillebø K, Holmen SD, Onsrud M, Gundersen SG, Taylor M, Kjetland EF, Ndung'U T. Effect of female genital schistosomiasis and anti-schistosomal treatment on monocytes, CD4+ T-Cells and CCR5 expression in the female genital tract. PLoS ONE. 2014; 9(6): e98593. doi: 10.1371/journal.pone.0098593

[17] Maizels RM, Bundy DAP, Selkirk ME, Smith DF, Anderson RM. Immunological modulation and evasion by helminth parasites in human populations. Nature. 1993; 365: 797–805.

[18] Janeway CA, Travers P, Walport M, Shlomchik M. Antigen presentation to lymphocytes. In: Schanck D, Austin P, Lawrence E, et al. editors, Immunobiology. The Immune System in Health and Disease. 5th ed. Chapters 1–14. T-Cell Mediated Immunity. Garland Publishing. Taylor and Francis Group, New York. 2001.

[19] Maizels RM, Balic A, Gomez-Escobar N, et al. Helminth parasites-Masters of regulation. Immunological Reviews. 2004; 201: 89–116.

[20] Bethony J, Brooker S, Albonico M, Geiger MS, Loukas A, Diemert D, Hotez PJ .Soil-transmitted helminth infections: ascariasis, trichuriasis, and hookworm. Lancet. 2006; 367: 1521–1532.

[21] Kalinkovinch A, Weisman Z, Greenberg Z, et al. Decreased CD4 and increased CD8 counts with T cell activation is associated with chronic helminth infection. Clinical and Experimental Immunology. 1998; 114: 414–421.

[22] Secor WE, Shah A, Mwinzi PMN, et al. Increased density of human immunodeficiency virus type 1 coreceptors CCR5 and CXCR4 on the surfaces of $CD4^+$ T cells and monocytes of patients with *Schistosoma mansoni* infection. Infection and Immunity. 2003; 71 (11): 6668–6671.

[23] Carrington M, O'Brien SJ. The influence of HLA genotype on AIDS. A seminal review that describes the association between HLA-A, HLA-B and HLA-C alleles and the rate of disease progression. Annual Review of Medicine. 2003; 54: 535–551.

[24] Liu R, et al. Homozygous defect in HIV-1 coreceptor accounts for resistance of some multiply-exposed individuals to HIV-1 infection. Cell. 1996; 86: 367–377.

[25] Schmitz JE, Kuroda MJ, Santra S, et al. Control of viremia in simian immunodeficiency virus infection by CD8+ lymphocytes. Science. 1999; 283: 857–860.

[26] Jin X, Bauer DE, Tuttleton SE, et al. Dramatic rise in plasma viremia after CD8+ T cell depletion in simian immunodeficiency virus-infected macaques. Journal of Experimental Medicine. 1999; 189: 991–998.

[27] Plummer FA, Ball TB, Kimani J, Fowke KR. Resistance to HIV-1 infection among highly exposed sex workers in Nairobi: what mediates protection and why does it develop? Immunology Letters. 1999; 66: 27–34.

[28] Ogg GS, Jin X, Bonhoeffer S, et al. Quantitation of HIV-1- specific cytotoxic T lymphocytes and plasma load of viral RNA. Science. 1998; 279: 2103–2106.

[29] McMichael AJ, Borrow P, Tomaras GD, Goonetilleke N, Haynes BF. The immune response during acute HIV-1 infection: clues for vaccine development. Nature Reviews Immunology. 2010; 10(1): 11–23. doi: 10.1038/nri2674

[30] Sousa AE, Carneiro J, Meier-Schellersheim M, et al. CD4 T cell depletion is linked directly to immune activation in the pathogenesis of HIV-1 and HIV-2 but only indirectly to the viral load. Journal of Immunology. 2002; 169: 3400–3406.

[31] Lu C-L, Murakowski DK, Bournazos S, Schoofs T, Sarkar D, Halper-Stromberg A, Horwitz JA, Nogueira L, Golijanin J, Gazumyan A, Ravetch JV, Caskey M, Chakraborty AK, Nussenzweig MC. Enhanced clearance of HIV-1-infected cells by broadly neutralizing antibodies against HIV-1 in vivo. Science. 2016. doi: 10.1126/science.aaf1279

[32] Joseph S, Jones FM, Laidlaw ME, Mohamed G, Mawa PA, Namujju PB, Kizza M, Watera C, Whitworth JA, Dunne DW, et al. Impairment of the Schistosoma mansoni-specific immune responses elicited by treatment with praziquantel in Ugandans with HIV-1 coinfection. Journal of Infectious Diseases. 2004; 190(3): 613–618.

[33] Maggi E, Mazzetti M, Ravina A, et al. Ability of HIV to promote a TH1 to TH0 shift and to replicate preferentially in TH2 and TH0 cells. Science. 1994; 265: 244–248.

[34] Lawn SD, Butera S, Folks TM. The contribution of immune activation to the pathogenesis and transmission of Human Immunodeficiency virus type1 infection. Clinical Microbiology Reviews. 2001; 14(4): 753–777.

[35] Henri S, Chevillard C, Mergani A, et al. Cytokine regulation of periportal fibrosis in humans infected with Schistosoma mansoni: IFN-γ is associated with protection against fibrosis and TNF-α with aggravation of disease. The Journal of Immunology. 2002; 169: 929–936.

[36] Ouaaz F, Ruscetti FW, Dugas B, MikovitsA J Agut H, Debre P, Mossalayi MD. Role of IgE immune complexes in the regulation of HIV-1 replication and increased cell death of infected Ul monocytes: involvement of CD23/FcdRII mediated nitric oxide and cyclic AMP pathways. Molecular Medicine. 1996; 2(1): 38–49.

[37] Lucey DR, Dorsky DI, Nicholson-Weller A, Weller PF. Human eosinophils express CD4 protein and bind human immunodeficiency virus gp120. The Journal of Experimental Medicine. 1989; 169: 327–332.

[38] Freedman AR, Gibson FM, Fleming SC, et al. Human immunodeficiency virus infection of eosinophils in human bone marrow cultures. The Journal of Experimental Medicine. 1991; 174: 1661–1664.

[39] Flynn JL, Chan J. Immunology of tuberculosis. Annual Review of Immunology. 2001; 19: 93–129.

[40] Rook GA, Dheda K, Zumla A. Immune responses to tuberculosis in developing countries: Implications for new vaccines. Nature Reviews Immunology. 2005; 5: 661–667.

[41] Kaufmann SH. Protection against tuberculosis: cytokines, T cells, and macrophages. Annals of the Rheumatic Diseases. 2002; 61: ii54–ii58.

[42] Giacomini E, Iona E, Ferroni L, Miettinen M, Fattorini L, Orefici G, Julkunen I, Coccia EM. Infection of human macrophages and dendritic cells with Mycobacterium tuberculosis induces a differential cytokine gene expression that modulates T cell response. Journal of Immunology. 2001; 166: 7033–7041.

[43] Cooper AM, Khader SA. The role of cytokines in the initiation, expansion, and control of cellular immunity to tuberculosis. Immunological Reviews. 2008; 226: 191–204.

[44] Trunz BB, Fine P, Dye C. Effect of BCG vaccination on childhood tuberculous meningitis and miliary tuberculosis worldwide: a meta-analysis and assessment of cost-effectiveness. The Lancet. 2006; 367: 1173–1180.

[45] Rafi W, Ribeiro-Rodrigues R, Ellner JJ, Salgame P. Coinfection-helminthes and tuberculosis. Current Opinion in HIV AIDS. 2012; 7(3): 239–244.

[46] Bentwich Z, Kalinkovich A, Weisman Z, Borkow G. Can eradication of helminthic infections change the face of AIDS and tuberculosis? Immunology Today. 1999; 20: 485–487.

[47] Flynn JL, Chan J. Tuberculosis: latency and reactivation. Infection and Immunity. 2001; 69(7): 4195–4201.

[48] Colditz GA, Brewer TF, Berkey CS, Wilson ME. Efficacy of BCG vaccine in the prevention of tuberculosis: meta-analysis of the published literature. Journal of the American Medical Association, 1994; 271: 698–702.

[49] Gandhi NR, Moll A, Sturm AW, Pawinski R, Govender T, Lalloo U, Zeller K, Andrews J, Friedland G. Extensively drug-resistant tuberculosis as a cause of death in patients co-infected with tuberculosis and HIV in a rural area of South Africa. Lancet. 2006; 368: 1575–1580.

[50] Babu S, Nutman TB. Helminth-tuberculosis co-infection: an immunologic perspective. Trends in Immunology. Elsevier Ltd; 2016; 37(9): 597–607.

[51] Horsnell W. How Helminths Alter Immunity to Infection in: Advances in Experimental Medicine and Biology 828, 2014. Chapter 3 and 6, Springer, New York. 1 p.

[52] Maizels RM, Yazdanbakhsh M. Immune regulation by helminth parasites: cellular and molecular mechanisms. Nature Reviews Immunology. 2003; 3: 733–744.

[53] Elias D, Wolday D, Akuffo H, Petros B, Bronner U, Britton S. Effect of deworming on human T cell responses to mycobacterial antigens in helminth-exposed individuals before and after bacille Calmette-Guérin (BCG) vaccination. Clinical & Experimental Immunology. 2001; 123: 219–225.

[54] Salgame P. Host innate and Th1 responses and the bacterial factors that control Mycobacterium tuberculosis infection. Current Opinion in Immunology. 2005; 17: 374–380. 24.

[55] Oldenhove G, de Heusch M, Urbain-Vansanten G, Urbain J, Maliszewski C, Leo O, Moser M. CD4+ CD25+ regulatory T cells control T helper cell type 1 responses to foreign antigens induced by mature dendritic cells in vivo. Journal of Experimental Medicine. 2003; 198: 259–266.

[56] Resende CT, Hirsch CS, Toossi Z, Dietze R, Ribeiro-Rodrigues R. Intestinal helminth co-infection has a negative impact on both anti-Mycobacterium tuberculosis immunity

and clinical response to tuberculosis therapy. Clinical & Experimental Immunology. 2007; 147: 45–52.

[57] van Soelen N, Mandalakas AM, Kirchner HL, Walzl G, Grewal HM, Jacobsen M, Hesseling AC. Effect of Ascaris Lumbricoides specific IgE on tuberculin skin test responses in children in a high-burden setting: a cross-sectional community-based study. BMC Infectious Diseases. 2012; 11(12): 211.

[58] Shapira-Nahor O, Kalinkovinch A, Weisman Z, et al. Increased susceptibility to HIV-1 infection of peripheral blood mononuclear cells from chronically immune-activated individuals. AIDS. 1998; 12: 1731–1733.

[59] Wolday D, Mayaan S, Mariam ZG, et al. Treatment of intestinal helminths is associated with decreased HIV plasma viral load. Journal of Acquired Immune Deficiency Syndromes. 2002; 31: 56–62.

[60] Elliot MA, Mawa PA, Joseph S, et al. Association between helminth infection and CD4+ T cell count, viral load and cytokine responses in HIV-1 infected Ugandan adults. Transactions of the Royal Society of Tropical Medicine and Hygiene. 2003; 97: 103–108.

[61] Gallagher M1, Malhotra I, Mungai PL, Wamachi AN, Kioko JM, Ouma JH, Muchiri E, King CL. The effects of maternal helminth and malaria infections on mother-to-child HIV transmission. AIDS. 2005; 19(16): 1849–1855.

[62] Kallestrup P, Zinyama R, Gomo E, et al. Schistosomiasis and HIV-1 infection in rural Zimbabwe: Effect of treatment of schistosomiasis on CD4 cell count and plasma HIV-1 RNA load. The Journal of Infectious Diseases. 2005; 192 (11): 1956–1961.

[63] Modjarrad K, Zulu I, Redden DT, Njobvu L, Lane HC, Bentwich Z, et al. Treatment of intestinal helminths does not reduce plasma concentrations of HIV-1 RNA in coinfected Zambian adults. Journal of Infectious Diseases [Internet]. 2005; 192(7): 1277–1283.

[64] Hosseinipour M, Napravnik S, Joaki G, et al. HIV and parasitic infection and the effect of treatment among adult outpatients in Malawi. The Journal of Infectious Diseases. 2007; 195: 1278–1282.

[65] Nielsen NO, Simonsen PE, Dalgaard P, Krarup H, Magnussen P, Magesa S, Friis H. Effect of diethylcarbamazine on HIV load, CD4%, and CD4/CD8 ratio in HIV-infected adult Tanzanians with or without lymphatic filariasis: randomized double-blind and placebo-controlled cross-over trial. American Journal of Tropical Medicine and Hygiene. 2007; 77: 507–513.

[66] Zinyama-Gutsire RBL, Chasela C, Madsen HO, Rusakaniko S, Kallestrup P, Christiansen M, Gomo E, Ullum H, Erikstrup C, Munyati S, Kurewa EN, Stray-Pedersen B, Garred P, Mduluza T. Role of Mannose-Binding Lectin Deficiency in HIV-1 and Schistosoma Infections in a Rural Adult Population in Zimbabwe. April 2015. PLoS ONE 10(4): e0122659. doi:10.1371/journal.pone.0122659

[67] Babatunde SK, Salami AK, Fabiyi JP, Agbede OO, Desalu OO. Prevalence of intestinal parasitic infestation in HIV seropositive and seronegative patients in Ilorin, Nigeria. Annals of African Medicine 2010; 9: 123–128.

[68] Walson JL, Otieno PA, Mbuchi M, Richardson BA, Lohman-Payne B, Macharia SW, Overbaugh J, Berkley J, Sanders EJ, Chung MH, John-Stewart GC. Albendazole treatment of HIV-1 and helminth co-infection: a randomized, double-blind, placebo-controlled trial. AIDS. 2008; 22(13): 1601–1609. doi: 10.1097/QAD.0b013e32830a502e.

[69] Akinbo FO, Okaka CE, Omoregie R. Prevalence of intestinal parasites in relation to CD4 counts and anaemia among HIV-infected patients in Benin City, Edo State, Nigeria. Tanzania Journal of Health Research. 2011; 13(1): 8–13.

[70] Jourdan PM, Holmen SD, Gundersen SG, Roald B, Kjetland EF. HIV target cells in Schistosoma haematobium-infected female genital mucosa. American Journal of Tropical Medicine and Hygiene. 2011; 85(6): 1060–1064. doi: 10.4269/ajtmh.2011.11-0135.

[71] Mkhize-KwitshanaZL, Taylor M, Jooste P, Mabaso MHL, Walzl G. The influence of different helminth infection phenotypes on immune responses against HIV in co-infected adults in South Africa. BMC Infectious Diseases 2011; 11: 273. http://www.biomedcentral.com/1471-2334/11/273.

[72] Idindili B. Challenges of continuum of HIV/AIDS care and treatment in Tanzania: The effects of parasites co-infections, HIV clinical manifestations, and adherence to antiretroviral therapy [doctoral dissertation] Basel: University of Basel; 2012. [cited 2016 Sept 13]. Available from: http://edoc.unibas.ch/22092/1/PhD_dissertation_Boniphace_Idindili.pdf

[73] Walson J, Singa B, Sangaré L, Naulikha J, Piper B, Richardson B, Otieno PA, Mbogo LW, Berkley JA, John-Stewart G. Empiric deworming to delay HIV disease progression in adults with HIV who are ineligible for initiation of antiretroviral treatment (the HEAT study): a multi-site, randomised trial. Lancet Infectious Diseases. 2012; 12(12): 925–932. doi: 10.1016/S1473-3099(12)70207-4.

[74] Webb EL, Kyosiimire-Lugemwa J, Kizito D, Nkurunziza P, Lule S, Muhangi L, Muwanga M, Kaleebu P, Elliott AM. The effect of anthelmintic treatment during pregnancy on HIV plasma viral load: results from a randomized, double-blind, placebo-controlled trial in Uganda. Journal of Acquired Immune Deficiency Syndromes. 2012; 60(3): 307–313. doi: 10.1097/QAI.0b013e3182511e42.

[75] Efraim M, Peck RN, Kalluvya SE, Kabangila R, Mazigo HD, Mpondo B, Bang H, Todd J, Fitzgerald DW, Downs JA. Schistosomiasis and impaired response to antiretroviral therapy among HIV-infected patients in Tanzania. Journal of Acquired Immune Deficiency Syndromes. 2013; 62(5): e153–e156. doi: 10.1097/QAI.0b013e318282a1a4.

[76] Mulu A, Maier M, Liebert UG. Deworming of intestinal helminths reduces HIV-1 subtype C viremia in chronically co-infected individuals. International Journal of Infectious Diseases 2013; 17(10): e897–e901.

[77] Gebreegziabiher D, Desta K, Desalegn G, Howe R, Abebe M. The effect of maternal helminth infection on maternal and neonatal immune function and immunity to tuberculosis. PLoS ONE. 2014; 9(4): e93429. doi: 10.1371/journal.pone.0093429

[78] Mkhize-Kwitshana ZL, Mabaso MLH, Walzl G. Proliferative capacity and cytokine production by cells of HIV-infected and uninfected adults with different helminth infection phenotypes in South Africa. BMC Infectious Diseases 2014; 14: 499.

[79] Lankowski AJ, Tsai AC, Kanyesigye M, Bwana M, Haberer JE, Wenger M, et al. Empiric deworming and CD4 count recovery in HIV-infected Ugandans initiating antiretroviral therapy. PLoS Neglected Tropical Diseases. 2014; 8(8): e3036. doi: 10.1371/journal.pntd.0003036

[80] Chachage M, Podola L, Clowes P, Nsojo A, Bauer A, Mgaya O, et al. Helminth-associated systemic immune activation and HIV co-receptor expression: response to albendazole/praziquantel treatment. PLoS Neglected Tropical Diseases. 3024; 8(3): e2755. doi: 10.1371/journal.pntd.0002755

[81] Noormahomed EV, Nhacupe N, Mascaró-Lazcano C, Mauaie MN, Buene T, Funzamo CA, et al. A cross-sectional serological study of cysticercosis, schistosomiasis, toxocariasis and echinococcosis in HIV-1 infected people in Beira, Mozambique. PLoS Neglected Tropical Diseases. 2014; 8(9): e3121.

[82] Abossie A, Petros B. Deworming and the immune status of HIV positive pre-antiretroviral therapy individuals in Arba Minch, Chencha and Gidole hospitals, Southern Ethiopia. BMC Research Notes. 2015; 8: 483. doi: 10.1186/s13104-015-1461-9.

[83] Kleppa E, Klinge KF, Galaphaththi-Arachchige HN, Holmen SD, Lillebø K, Onsrud M, et al. Schistosoma haematobium infection and CD4+ T-cell levels: a cross-sectional study of young South African women. PLoS ONE. 2015; 10(3): e0119326. doi: 10.1371/journal.pone.0119326

[84] Mengist HM, Taye B, Tsegaye A. Intestinal parasitosis in relation to CD4+T cells levels and anemia among HAART initiated and HAART naive pediatric HIV patients in a model ART center in Addis Ababa, Ethiopia. PLoS ONE. 2015; 10(2): e0117715. doi: 10.1371/journal.pone.0117715

[85] Mulu A, Anagaw B, Gelaw A, Ota F, Kassu A, Yifru S. Effect of deworming on Th2 immune response during HIV-helminths co-infection. Journal of Translational Medicine. 2015; 13: 236. doi: 10.1186/s12967-015-0600-3

[86] Malhotra I, Mungai P, Wamachi A, Kioko J, Ouma JH, et al. Helminth- and bacillus Calmette-Guerin-induced immunity in children sensitized in utero to filariasis and schistosomiasis. Journal of Immunology. 1999; 162: 6843–6848.

[87] Adams JF, Schölvinck EH, Gie RP, Potter PC, Beyers N, Beyers AD. Decline in total serum IgE after treatment for tuberculosis. Lancet. 1999; 353(9169): 2030–2033.

[88] Stewart GR, Boussinesq M, Coulson T, Elson L, Nutman T, et al. Onchocerciasis modulates the immune response t mycobacterial antigens. Clinical & Experimental Immunology. 1999; 117: 517–523.

[89] Elliott, AM, Kyosiimire J, Quigley MA, Nakiyingi J, Watera C, Brown M, Joseph S, French N, Gilks CF, Withworth JAG. Eosinophilia and progression to active tuberculosis in HIV-1-infected Ugandans. Transactions of the Royal Society of Tropical Medicine and Hygiene. 2003; 97: 477–480.

[90] Kassu A, Tsegaye A, Wolday D, et al. Role of incidental and/or cured intestinal parasitic infections on profile of CD4+ and CD8+ T-cell subsets and activation status in HIV-1 infected and uninfected adult Ethiopians. Clinical & Experimental Immunology. 2003; 132: 113–119.

[91] Kassu A, Mohammad A, Fujimaki Y, Moges F, Elias D, Mekonnen F, Mengistu G, Yamato M, Wondmikun Y, Ota F. Serum IgE levels of tuberculosis patients in a tropical setup with high prevalence of HIV and intestinal parasitoses. Clinical & Experimental Immunology. 2004; 138(1): 122–127.

[92] Elias D, Mengistu G, Akuffo H, Britton S. Are intestinal helminths risk factors for developing active tuberculosis? Tropical Medicine & International Health. 2006; 11: 551–558.

[93] Elias D, Britton S, Aseffa A, Engers H, Akuffo H. Poor immunogenicity of BCG in helminth infected population is associated with increased in vitro TGF-beta production. Vaccine. 2008; 26: 3897–3902.

[94] Webb EL, Mawa PA, Ndibazza J, et al. Effect of single-dose anthelmintic treatment during pregnancy on an infant's response to immunisation and on susceptibility to infectious diseases in infancy: a randomised, double-blind, placebo-controlled trial. Lancet. 2011; 377: 52–62.

[95] Wassie L, Aseffa A, Abebe M, et al. Parasitic infection may be associated with discordant responses to QuantiFERON and tuberculin skin test in apparently healthy children and adolescents in a tuberculosis endemic setting, Ethiopia. BMC Infectious Diseases. 2013; 13: 265.

[96] Biraro IA, Egesa M, Toulza F, Levin J, Cose S, Joloba M, et al. Impact of co-infections and BCG immunisation on immune responses among household contacts of tuberculosis patients in a Ugandan cohort. PLoS ONE. 2014; 9(11): e111517.

[97] Abate E, Belayneh M, Idh J, Diro E, Elias D, Britton S, et al. Asymptomatic helminth infection in active tuberculosis is associated with increased regulatory and Th-2 responses and a lower sputum smear positivity. PLoS Neglected Tropical Diseases. 2015; 9(8): e00039.

[98] Abate E, Belayneh M, Gelaw A, Idh J, Getachew A, Alemu S, et al. The impact of asymptomatic helminth co-infection in patients with newly diagnosed tuberculosis in North-West Ethiopia. PLoS ONE. 2012; 7(8): e42901.

[99] Cooper PJ, Chico ME, Sandoval C, et al. Human infection with Ascaris lumbricoides is associated with suppression of the interleukin-2 response to recombinant cholera toxin B subunit following vaccination with the live oral cholera vaccine CVD 103-HgR. Infection and Immunity. 2001; 69(3): 1574–1580.

[100] Cooper PJ, Chico ME, Losonsky G, et al. Albendazole treatment of children with ascariasis enhances the vibriocidal antibody response to the live attenuated oral cholera vaccine CVD 103-HgR. The Journal of Infectious Diseases. 2000; 182: 1199–1206.

[101] Cooper PJ, Espinel I, Parades W, et al. Impaired tetanus-specific cellular and humoral responses following tetanus vaccination in human onchocerciais: a possible role for interleukin -10. The Journal of Infectious Diseases. 1998; 178(4): 1133–1138.

[102] Kroidl I, Saathoff E, Maganga L, Makunde WH, Hoerauf A, Geldmacher C, Clowes P, Maboko L, Hoelscher M. Effect of Wuchereria bancrofti infection on HIV incidence in southwest Tanzania: a prospective cohort study. Lancet. 2016; pii: S0140-6736(16) 31252-1. doi: 10.1016/S0140-6736(16)31252-1.

[103] Gopinath R, Ostrowski M, Justement SJ, et al. Filarial infections increase susceptibility to human immunodeficiency virus infection in peripheral blood mononuclear cells in vitro. The Journal of Infectious Diseases. 2000; 182: 1804–1808.

[104] Rizardi GP, Harari A, Capiluppi B, Tambussi G, Ellefsen K, Ciuffreda D, et al. Treatment of primary HIV-1 infection with cyclosporin A coupled with highly active antiretroviral therapy. Journal of Clinical Investigation. 2002; 109(5): 681–688.

[105] Means A, Burns P, Sinclair D, Walson JL. Antihelminthics in helminth endemic areas: effects on HIV infection. Cochrane Database of Systematic Reviews. 2016, Issue 4. Art. No.: CD006419. doi: 10.1002/14651858.CD006419.pub4.Accessed 2016-08-29.

[106] Guadalupe I, Mitre E, Benitez S, Chico ME, Nutman TB, Cooper PJ. Evidence for in utero sensitization to Ascaris lumbricoides in newborns of mothers with ascariasis. Journal of Infectious Diseases. 2009; 199: 01846–1850.

Chapter 5

Atherosclerosis and Helminths Infection

Shi-Wei Shen, Yun Lu, Feng Li, Zhen-Hai Shen, Ming Xu, Wei-Feng Yao, Hua-Jin Qi, Ling Zhou, Yin-Bo Feng, Ling Wang, Jing-Ting Yun and Da-Xin Tong

Additional information is available at the end of the chapter

http://dx.doi.org/10.5772/65515

Abstract

Atherosclerosis is a chronic disease that causes various cardiovascular complications. Plaque formation in atherosclerosis is considered similar to the pathogenesis of other autoimmune diseases; thus, immunomodulation and immunosuppression may present strategies for the treatment and prevention of these diseases. Interestingly helminth infection was found to inhibit T helper 1-mediated autoimmune diseases and T helper 2-mediated allergy and asthma, indicating significant potential for clinical application. Some study even found that therapeutic efficacy of the viable tapeworm was superior to dexamethasone treatment. Recently, some studies have shown an inverse association between helminth infections and inflammatory diseases, including diabetes mellitus, lipid abnormality, and atherosclerosis. Will the underlying mechanism bring us a new idea on the treatment for these diseases? We tried to find an answer by reviewing recent articles.

Keywords: previous helminth infection, cardiovascular diseases risk factors, negative regulation of immune response

1. Introduction

Atherosclerosis is a chronic disease that causes artery walls to thicken and become less elastic. The consequent restriction of blood flow can cause various problems such as heart attacks, stroke, renal failure, and other serious cardiovascular complications. In general, the suscept-ibility to atherosclerosis depends on diabetes, hypertension, high cholesterol, hyperhomocysteinemia, genetic factors, diet, smoking, and lack of exercise. In addition, some studies consider that inflammation and immunity are central to atherosclerosis onset [1, 2].

Interestingly, helminths infection is regarded not only as an infectious disease but also as an immunological disease. Helminth antigen has been shown to induce metabonomic changes and to mediate the host autoimmune response [3].

Helminth infection was also found to inhibit T helper 1 (Th1)-mediated autoimmune diseases and T helper 2 (Th2)-mediated allergy and asthma, indicating a significant potential for clinical application [4–10].

Some study even found that therapeutic efficacy of the viable tapeworm was superior to dexamethasone treatment [6].

Will the recent findings of the underlying mechanism on the inverse association between helminth infections and inflammatory diseases, including diabetes mellitus, lipid abnormality, and atherosclerosis, bring us a new idea on the treatment for these diseases? Now, let us go and review these interesting studies.

2. The relationship between helminth infections and diabetes mellitus

Diabetes is a chronic metabolic disease. It is characterized by elevated blood glucose levels caused by insufficient insulin production from β-islet cells of the pancreas, or impaired insulin sensitivity of insulin target organs. The number of people with diabetes mellitus is increasing worldwide. As reported by International Diabetes Federation, around 387 million people were living with diabetes in 2014. It is predicted that in 2035 up to 592 million will suffer from diabetes. At present, diabetes mellitus has been found in 8.3% of adults, and China is a major site of this rapidly emerging epidemic.

Inflammatory immune responses play a crucial role in the progression of β-islet cell destruction in both type 1 (T1D) and type 2 diabetes (T2D). As shown above, a strong predictor for the development of type 2 diabetes mellitus (T2D) is insulin resistance. Inflammation and altered innate immunity have also been implicated in the pathogenesis of diabetes through insulin resistance.

Conversely, helminth infections are well known to affect the metabolic profiles and risk of diabetes by inducing type 2 and anti-inflammatory immune responses that are able to modulate the activity of the innate immune response [11, 12].

Both experimental and epidemiological studies reported such a beneficial impact of helminth infections on T1D and more recently on T2D.

Schramm et al. [13] have shown that *Schistosoma mansoni* infections can adopt an immune evasion strategy by inducing regulatory T cells, which in turn may decrease systemic inflammation and the development of inflammatory diseases, including diabetes.

Paola et al. [14] found infection with *S. mansoni* or exposure to eggs from this helminth inhibits the development of type 1 diabetes in NOD mice. The host responses normally induced by infection with *S. mansoni* or exposure to its antigens enable peripheral tolerance to β-cell antigens. Effects on the innate immune system may therefore deviate T-cell responses to the pancreatic beta cell towards a benign Th2 response but also influence the development of regulatory T cells.

Hussaarts [15] found that chronic helminth infection and helminth-derived molecules protect against metabolic disorders by promoting the Th2 response, eosinophilia, and WAT M2 polarization. Helminth parasites are the strongest natural inducers of type 2 immune responses, and short-lived infection with rodent nematodes was reported to improve glucose tolerance in obese mice. That is to say, chronic helminth infection and helminth-derived egg antigens promote adipose tissue M2 macrophages and improve insulin sensitivity in obese mice.

A cross-sectional study has been conducted on the basis of human being, in Jiading, a suburb of Shanghai [16]; it reported that previous helminth infection might reduce the prevalence of diabetes and metabolic syndrome.

Apparently, helminths infection can also reduce energy intake and thereby change the energy balance, which may be another beneficial in terms of insulin resistance [17].

At a molecular level, mTOR, a serine/threonine protein kinase, which is located downstream of insulin signaling, plays an essential role in immune cell energy metabolism and function [18]. Moreover, it has been shown that STAT6 signaling downstream of IL-4, as well as Th2 responses induced by helminths, has the capacity to improve glucose metabolism and insulin signaling [19].

In humans, immune intervention with IL-1 receptor antagonist (Anakinra) has also been shown to influence glucose metabolism [20].

A recent study by Locksley and colleagues [3] has demonstrated elegantly that helminth-induced adipose tissue eosinophilia enhanced glucose tolerance and improved insulin resistance in mice fed a high-fat diet. Moreover, although the parasite was cleared after 8 days, metabolic response was sustained.

Both epidemiological and experimental studies indicate that helminths may be able to ameliorate obesity-induced insulin resistance. The ongoing SUGARSPIN trial investigates the association of helminth infections with insulin sensitivity and the effect of anti-helminth treatment on insulin sensitivity in Indonesia, which will help to further decipher the impact of helminth infection on glucose homeostasis [21].

Type 2 and regulatory immune responses induced by helminths accompanied by increases in alternatively activated macrophages, anti-inflammatory cytokines and regulatory T cells present possible protective mechanisms to attenuate autoimmune responses in diet-induced insulin resistance in T2D and T1D. In addition to infections with living helminths, administrations of helminth-derived products have also played a role in protecting against both T1D and T2D in animal models. Hence, helminths and their products may provide new treatment strategies for diabetes [22].

3. The relationship between helminth infections and lipid abnormalities

Generally, dyslipidemia characterized by hypertriglyceridemia and low HDL-C is called "atherogenic dyslipidemia." This disorder may increase the concentration of triglyceride-rich lipoprotein (TRL) and its remnants, accelerate the inflammatory reaction in the arterial wall, and aggravate the damage to endothelial cells [23]. Elevated TRL may result in an increase in small, dense LDL (sdLDL), which exerts a strong atherogenic action, and in a reduction in HDL-C, which is involved in reverse cholesterol transport [24]. Moreover, TRL remnants are deposited in the arterial wall, thereby promoting atherosclerosis [25]. Recently, this dyslipidemia was identified as a residual cardiovascular risk factor following the reduction in LDL-C by statin treatment [26]. Dyslipidemia has also been found in patients with systemic lupus erythematosus (SLE) and rheumatoid arthritis (RA) [27].

Stanley [28] provide an evidence that the serum cholesterol-lowering effect is mediated by factors released from *S. mansoni* eggs and that high levels of lipids, particularly triacylglycerols and cholesteryl esters, present in the uninfected livers of both random-bred and apoE(−/−) mice fed a high-fat diet were not present in livers of the helminth-infected mice.

Our studies also indicate that the potential long-term effects of previous helminth infection may improve the blood lipid metabolism (reduction in TG and elevation of HDL-C) and reduce the atherogenic index of plasma [29–31]. Another study also found significantly lower plasma lipid levels in children (aged 7–13Â years) infected with *Schistosoma haematobium* compared with controls ($p < 0.01$) (http://www.pakmedinet.com). Recent studies in rural Indonesia showed that intestinal helminth infections were negatively associated with lipid levels [4, 32–35].

Magen et al. [36] reported in an autopsy study that *Opisthorchis felineus* chronic helminthic infections was found to be associated with lower serum total cholesterol levels and a significant attenuation of atherosclerosis.

One of the possible mechanisms of helminth anti-atherosclerotic action might be a disorder in the liver function after helminth infection, resulted in a decrease in the synthetic ability of the liver, which reduce its production of cholesterol.

Another mechanism of lipid lowering in the host might be a direct uptake of lipids by flat worms or as an alteration in the uptake of lipids by the host. Parasites are able to remodel host lipids for their growth [37]. They have developed unique metabolic pathways that allow them to survive and multiply by scavenging nutrients from the host [38].

Additionally, immune modulation causing Th2 polarization can change lipid metabolism; total plasma cholesterol levels were found to be increased in Th1 polarized, IL-4-deficient or STAT-6-deficient mice [39, 40].

4. The relationship between helminth infections and atherosclerosis

Plaque formation in atherosclerosis is considered similar to the pathogenesis of other autoimmune diseases; thus, immunomodulation and immunosuppression may present strategies for the treatment and prevention of these diseases [41].

Parasitic helminths have coexisted with human beings throughout time. Success in eradicating helminths has limited helminth-induced morbidity and mortality but is also correlated with increasing rates of "Western" diseases, including atherosclerosis [42].

The immune response induced by helminth infection is an important host defense mechanism against pathogens. Specific immune pathways, such as modified type-2 responses, induced by helminthes have been implicated in protective host responses to homoeostatic perturbations, such as metabolic dysfunction and atherosclerosis [43].

A preventive injection of soluble egg antigen (SEA) of *S. japonicum* to ApoE/mice has also displayed anti-atherosclerosis activity by increasing the proportion of CD4+CD25+ regulatory T (Treg) cells and inhibiting inflammatory cytokine production in the early stage of the disease [44]. This alleviated the immunopathological injury to the host liver and directly inhibited the host immune response to infections, which help the antigen escape from host immunity [45]. Treg cells exert an immunosuppressive function which is very important in the maintenance of immune homeostases and immune tolerance [46].

Subramanian et al. [47] also reported that the immune system can develop resistance to atherosclerotic lesions and the anti-inflammatory T-cell effect produced by the immune system may help inhibit the progression of atherosclerosis. Helminth antigens have been found to induce metabonomic alterations and mediate the host immune response, which produce a strong anti-inflammatory response to help suppress the development of arteriosclerosis in mice.

A negative correlation between a helminth, Schistosoma infection, and the risk of cardiovascular disease has been reported both in the past and at present [31, 48]. Helminths are eukaryotic parasitic worms, which induce a Th2 response and alternatively activate macrophages that are crucial for host survival. After *S. mansoni* infection, a higher expression of alternative macrophage markers is observed [49]. The *S. mansoni*-derived soluble egg antigens (SEA) have been reported as new modulators of the macrophage phenotype in vivo [50]. Indeed, plaque size of LDLR−/− mice reduced after SEA treatment, with the reduction in cholesterol content in lesion, decreased expression of inflammatory markers [51].

The dendritic cells (DCs) are able to prime strong Th2 responses that indicated these cells are also an attractive target for therapeutic manipulation of the immune system in the context of metabolic disorders. As DCs have the capacity of regulating a wide array of T-cell responses, they are widely studied as targets for development of vaccines and immunotherapies [52–54]. Therapeutic manipulation of DCs might also provide a new strategy for targeted treatment of atherosclerosis [55].

Further studies to investigate the exact mechanisms underlying immunomodulation and immunosuppression in previous helminth infection and the likelihood of schistosomiasis vaccines to inhibit atherosclerosis development seem justified.

Acknowledgements

The research reported in this article was supported by Jiangsu Department of Health, China (Grant Nos.: BJ15032, BJ15033, Y2015073, Z201519, BJ14023, and B2013073.), the R & D Fund of Wuxi Municipal Science & Technology Bureau, China (Grant No.: CMB21S1301), the Natural Science Foundation of Jiangsu Province, China (Grant Nos.: BK20151115, BK20131096, and BK2011162,) and the National Natural Science Foundation of China (Grant No.: 81600346).

Author details

Shi-Wei Shen[1,4], Yun Lu[2,4], Feng Li[2,4], Zhen-Hai Shen[2,4*], Ming Xu[3], Wei-Feng Yao[1], Hua-Jin Qi[2], Ling Zhou[2], Yin-Bo Feng[2], Ling Wang[2], Jing-Ting Yun[2] and Da-Xin Tong[2]

*Address all correspondence to: shentaihu@126.com

1 Wuxi No. 2 People's Hospital Affiliated to Nanjing Medical University, Wuxi, Jiangsu, China

2 Jiangsu Provincial Taihu Cadre's Sanatorium of Jiangsu Provincial People's Hospital Group, Wuxi, Jiangsu, China

3 Jiangsu Institute of Parasitic Diseases, Wuxi, Jiangsu, China

4 Co-first authors.

References

[1] Ohashi R, Mu H, Yao Q, Chen C. Atherosclerosis: immunopathogenesis and immunotherapy. Med Sci Monit. 2004;10:255–260.

[2] Mahmoudi M, Curzen N, Gallagher PJ. Atherogenesis: the role of inflammations and infection. Histopathology 2007;50:535–546.

[3] Wu D, Molofsky AB, Liang HE, et al. Eosinophils sustain adipose alternatively activated macrophages associated with glucose homeostasis. Science 2011;332:243–247.

[4] Adult Treatment Panel III. Third Report of the National Cholesterol Education Program (NCEP) Expert Panel on Detection, Evaluation, and Treatment of High Blood Cholesterol in Adults (Adult Treatment Panel III) final report. Circulation 2002;106:3143–3421.

[5] Adisakwattana P, Saunders SP, Nel HJ, et al. Helminth-derived immunomodulatory molecules. Adv Exp Med Biol. 2009;666:95–107.

[6] Melon A, Wang A, Phan V, McKay DM. Infection with *Hymenolepis diminuta* is more effective than daily corticosteroids in blocking chemically induced colitis in mice. J Biomed Biotechnol. 2010;2010:384523.

[7] Osada Y, Shimizu S, Kumagai T, et al. *Schistosoma mansoni* infection reduces severity of collagen-induced arthritis via downregulation of pro-inflammatory mediators. Int J Parasitol. 2009;39:457–464.

[8] Bager P, Arnved J, Roslash;nborg S, et al. *Trichuris suis* ova therapy for allergic rhinitis: a randomized, double blind, placebo-controlled clinical trial. J Allergy Clin Immunol. 2010;125:123–130.

[9] Zaccone P, Burton OT, Cooke A. Interplay of parasite-driven immune responses and autoimmunity. Trends Parasitol. 2008;24:35–42.

[10] Osada Y, Kanazawa T. Parasitic helminths: new weapons against immunological disorders. J Biomed Biotechnol. 2010;2010:743758.

[11] Wellen KE, Hotamisligil GS. Inflammation, stress, and diabetes. J Clin Invest. 2005;115:1111–1119.

[12] Thabet HS, Saleh NK, Thabet SS, Abdel-Aziz M, Kalleny NK. Decreased basal non-insulin-stimulated glucose uptake by diaphragm in streptozotocin-induced diabetic mice infected with *Schistosoma mansoni*. Parasitol Res. 2008;103:595–601.

[13] Schramm G, Haas H. Th2 immune response against *Schistosoma mansoni* infection. Microbes Infect. 2010;12:881–888.

[14] Zaccone P, Fehervari Z, Jones FM, et al. *Schistosoma mansoni* antigens modulate the activity of the innate immune response and prevent onset of type 1 diabetes. Eur J Immunol. 2003;33:1439–1449.

[15] Hussaarts L, García-Tardón N, van Beek L, et al. Chronic helminth infection and helminth-derived egg antigens promote adipose tissue M2 macrophages and improve insulin sensitivity in obese mice. FASEB J. 2015;29(7):3027–3039.

[16] Chen Y, Lu J, Huang Y, et al. Association of previous Helminths infection with diabetes and metabolic syndrome: a cross-sectional study in rural China. J Clin Endocrinol Metab. 2013;98:E283–E287.

[17] Papier K, Williams GM, Luceres-Catubig R, et al. Childhood malnutrition and parasitic helminth interactions. Clin Infect Dis. 2014;59:234–243.

[18] Fox CJ, Hammerman PS, Thompson CB. Fuel feeds function: energy metabolism and the T-cell response. Nat Rev Immunol. 2005;5:844–852.

[19] Ricardo-Gonzalez RR, Red EA, Odegaard JI, et al. IL-4/STAT6 immune axis regulates peripheral nutrient metabolism and insulin sensitivity. Proc Natl Acad Sci USA. 2010;107:22617–22622.

[20] van Asseldonk EJ, Stienstra R, Koenen TB, et al. Treatment with Anakinra improves disposition index but not insulin sensitivity in nondiabetic subjects with the metabolic syndrome: a randomized, double-blind, placebo-controlled study. J Clin Endocrinol Metab. 2011;96:2119–2126.

[21] Tahapary DL, de Ruiter K, Martin et al. Helminth infections and type 2 diabetes: a cluster-randomized placebo controlled SUGARSPIN trial in Nangapanda, Flores, Indonesia. BMC Infect Dis. 2015;15:133.

[22] Berbudi A, Ajendra J, Wardani AP, et al. Parasitic helminths and their beneficial impact on type 1 and type 2 diabetes. Diabetes Metab Res Rev. 2016;32:238–250.

[23] Wang L, Gill R, Pedersen TL, et al. Triglyceride-rich lipoprotein lipolysis releases neutral and oxidized FFAs that induce endothelial cell inflammation. Lipid Res. 2009;50:204–213.

[24] Berneis KK, Krauss RM. Metabolic origins and clinical significance of LDL heterogeneity. Lipid Res. 2002;43:1363–1379.

[25] Mangat R, Su JW, Lambert JE, et al. Increased risk of cardiovascular disease in Type 1 diabetes: arterial exposure to remnant lipoproteins leads to enhanced deposition of cholesterol and binding to glycated extracellular matrix proteoglycans. Diabetic Med. 2011;28:61–72.

[26] Miller M. Is hypertriglyceridemia an independent risk factor for coronary heart disease? The epidemiological evidence. Eur Heart J. 1998;19(Suppl H):H18–H22.

[27] Sherer Y, Zinger H, Shoenfeld Y. Atherosclerosis in systemic lupus erythematosus. Autoimmunity 2010;43:98–102.

[28] Stanley RG, Jackson CL, Griffiths K, et al. Effects of *Schistosoma mansoni* worms and eggs on circulating cholesterol and liver lipids in mice. Atherosclerosis 2009;207(1): 131–138.

[29] Shen SW, Lu Y, Shen ZH, et al. The potential long-term effect of previous Helminths infection reduces the risk of metabolic syndrome among Chinese men. Parasite Immunol. 2015;37:333–339.

[30] Shen SW, Lu Y, Shen ZH, et al. Potential long-term effects of previous Helminths infection may reduce the atherogenic index of plasma in Chinese men. Int J Parasitol. 2015;45:289–294.

[31] Shen SW, Lu Y, Shen ZH, et al. The potential long-term effect of previous schistosome infection may reduce the risk factors for cardiovascular diseases. Int J Parasitol. 2014;177:566–568.

[32] Wiria AE, Djuardi Y, Supali T, et al. Helminth infection in populations undergoing epidemiological transition: a friend or foe? Semin Immunopathol. 2012;34:889–901.

[33] Wiria AE, Wammes LJ, Hamid F, et al. Relationship between carotid intima media thickness and helminth infections on Flores Island, Indonesia. PLoS One 2013;8:e54855.

[34] Pasha SM, Wiria AE, Wammes LJ, et al. Blood pressure class and carotid artery intima-media thickness in a population at the secondary epidemiological transition. J Hypertens. 2011;29:2194–2200.

[35] Wiria AE, Sartono E, Supali T, et al. Helminth infections, type-2 immune response, and metabolic syndrome. PLoS Pathog. 2014;10:e1004140.

[36] Magen E, Bychkov V, Ginovker A, et al. Chronic *Opisthorchis felineus* infection attenuates atherosclerosis--an autopsy study. Int J Parasitol. 2013;43:819–824.

[37] Bansal D, Bhatti HS, Sehgal R. Role of cholesterol in parasitic infections. Lipids Health Dis. 2005;9:10.

[38] Das S, Stevens T, Castillo C, et al. Lipid metabolism in mucous-dwelling amitochondriate protozoa. Int J Parasitol. 2002;32:655–657.

[39] Huber SA, Sakkinen P, David C, et al. T helper-cell phenotype regulates atherosclerosis in mice under conditions of mild hypercholesterolemia. Circulation 2001;103:2610–2616.

[40] King VL, Szilvassy SJ, Daugherty A. Interleukin-4 deficiency promotes gallstone formation. J Lipid Res. 2002;43:768–771.

[41] Hansson GK. Inflammation, atherosclerosis, and coronary artery disease. N Engl J Med. 2005;352:1685–1695.

[42] Guigas B, Molofsky AB. A worm of one's own: how helminths modulate host adipose tissue function and metabolism. Trends Parasitol. 2015;31:435–441.

[43] von Moltke J, Locksley RM. I-L-C-2 it: type 2 immunity and group 2 innate lymphoid cells in homeostasis. Curr Opin Immunol. 2014;31C:58–65.

[44] Zhang H, Xing Y, Kong H, et al. Anti-atherogenic effect and its mechanisms of soluble egg antigen of *Schistosomia japonicum* in ApoE mice. Chin J Schisto Control. 2012;24:654–658.

[45] McKay DM. The therapeutic helminth? Trends Parasitol. 2009;25:109–114.

[46] Mueller DL. Mechanism maintaining peripheral tolerance. Nat Immunol. 2010;11:21–27.

[47] Subramanian M, Thorp E, Hansson GK, Tabas I. Treg-mediated suppression of atherosclerosis requires MYD88 signaling in DCs. J Clin Invest. 2013;123:179–188.

[48] Assaad-Khalil SH, Lachine N, Sidrak M, et al. Immuno-metabolic factors in schistosomal hepatic fibrosis modulating atherogenesis. Ann Biol Clin (Paris). 1992;50:697–701.

[49] Cudejko C, Wouters K, Fuentes L, et al. p16INK4a deficiency promotes IL-4-induced polarization and inhibits proinflammatory signaling in macrophages. Blood 2011;118:2556–2566.

[50] Wolfs IM, Stoger JL, Goossens P, et al. Reprogramming macrophages to an anti-inflammatory phenotype by helminth antigens reduces murine atherosclerosis. FASEB J. 2014;28:288–299.

[51] De Paoli F, Staels B, Chinetti-Gbaguidi G. Macrophage phenotypes and their modulation in atherosclerosis. Circ J. 2014;78:1775–1781.

[52] Steinman RM. Dendritic cells in vivo: a key target for a new vaccine science. Immunity 2008;29:319–324.

[53] Palucka K, Banchereau J. Cancer immunotherapy via dendritic cells. Nat Rev Cancer. 2012;12:265–277.

[54] Thomson AW, Robbins PD. Tolerogenic dendritic cells for autoimmune disease and transplantation. Ann Rheum Dis. 2008;67:iii90–iii96.

[55] Hussaarts L, Yazdanbakhsh M, Guigas B. Priming dendritic cells for th2 polarization: lessons learned from helminths and implications for metabolic disorders. Front Immunol. 2014;20:499.

Section 4

Therapy and Preventive Measures

Chapter 6

Global Control Efforts of Schistosomiasis and Soil-Transmitted Helminthiasis

Takafira Mduluza, Tawanda J. Chisango,
Agness F. Nhidza and Amos Marume

Additional information is available at the end of the chapter

http://dx.doi.org/10.5772/65282

Abstract

Schistosomiasis is a waterborne disease whose life cycle involves freshwater sources conducive for the survival and reproduction of aquatic snails that form a connective link between man and water in the life cycle and transmission of schistosomiasis. The African region has network of rivers with freshwater suggesting the presence of schistosomiasis and difficulty to control. Some communities, due to socioeconomic challenges, have inadequate sanitation and water supply; use of bush toilets for excretion is commonly practiced. These conditions in Africa also promote transmission of soil-transmitted helminthiasis. The World Health Organization (WHO), in response to the public health and socioeconomic impact of neglected tropical diseases, is coordinating strategies for the control and elimination of the diseases including schistosomiasis and soil-transmitted helminthiasis. As one of the milestones, mapping of neglected tropical diseases in the African region has been prioritized for the implementation of control strategies. In countries where mapping has been completed, WHO and its partners are supplying medicines required for annual mass treatment for preventive chemotherapy and encourage countries to take ownership in implementing complementary strategies for morbidity control, elimination and eradication of country-specific neglected tropical diseases. The mainstay of helminthiasis control is preventive chemotherapy, targeting school age children to prevent morbidity and development of pathological manifestations, including urogenital schistosomiasis that is understood to contribute to HIV transmission. Vaccines are still to be discovered and designed, with many possible antigen candidates, but however the immune responses are still to be fully understood. There is need to understand the subtle link between each component of the immune responses and the host immunogenetics impacting on the translated immunological response of cytokines that are delicately controlled for cellular immunity and antibody production. Currently, preventive chemotherapy treatment is the only control method in concert with health education in an attempt to cut the helminthiasis life cycle.

Keywords: control, schistosomiasis, soil-transmitted helminthiasis, mass drug administration, chemotherapy

1. Introduction

Parasitic worms (helminths) are responsible for chronic infections of over two billion people worldwide and impose a huge public health burden. The hallmark of helminth infection is immune modulation of the host's immune response, which both limits immunopathology in the host while allowing the worms to evade host immune attack. The immune modulation of host responses during helminth infection has attracted much interest in terms to understand the generation of protective immunity. Unfortunately, the immune modulation occurring during helminth infection also interferes with the expression of naturally acquired protective immunity against the parasites, resulting in an accumulation of parasites in the host. Experimental Studies suggest manipulating host regulatory responses can enhance helminths vaccine efficacy. In human schistosomiasis, the health impact is not confined to immunopathology but extends to physical damage resulting from the presence of the parasites and the passage of parasite eggs as they are excreted from the host via urine or stool. In the case of urogenital schistosomiasis, infection interferes with child development and health, diminishes female reproductive health and increases susceptibility to sexually transmitted diseases including HIV and can lead to bladder cancer.

Currently available control method is treatment of infected people with the antihelminthic drug praziquantel. Field studies have already demonstrated that praziquantel treatment can induce protective immunity in chronically infected children, while treatment if conducted earlier in life would mean children benefit from the effects of praziquantel earlier, thus avoiding the health costs associated with chronic infections. Praziquantel treatment imparts on molecular and immune responses, mediating resistance in individuals previously with chronic schistosome who became resistant against reinfection by the parasites. This concept of infection-treatment as immunization is used in some veterinary diseases. There is need to investigate the transcriptional and post-translational characteristics underlying resistance to schistosome. Subsequently, regular childhood treatment may induce protective immune responses, that is, treatment of primary infections before it becomes chronic, induces regulatory responses that may reduce the efficacy of the effector responses. More studies are required to understand the activation of regulatory, pro- and anti-inflammatory responses in individuals who remain susceptible to re-infection and the mechanisms by which these regulatory responses modulate effector functions. Such knowledge is important to improving current and future helminth interventions as well as the development of novel therapeutics against immune-mediated pathology arising from parasitic infection or immune dysfunction.

An important constraint for helminths vaccine development is the paucity of information on the induction of appropriate effector pathways mediating protective immunity over the regulatory responses, which modulate them, as well as on mechanisms by which vaccine efficacy and longevity can be enhanced. Experimental studies of other helminths suggest that vaccine efficacy can be improved beyond the typical low protection level by neutralizing immunomodulatory processes. There is missing evidence to identify the key immunomodulators and their functional mechanisms, which can be manipulated to improve the efficacy of helminths vaccines and pathways that can be manipulated to enhance the longevity of vaccine-induced resistance. In addition, there is currently lack of consensus on markers of vaccine-induced protection. However, in the meantime, preventive chemotherapy is the only alternative in concert with health education.

1.1. Human helminthiasis as neglected tropical diseases

Human helminthiasis are part of the neglected tropical diseases (NTDs), which are a diverse group of parasitic, viral and bacterial diseases with distinct characteristics, that thrive mainly among the poorest populations, hinder socioeconomic development and cause substantial illness for more than one billion people globally [1]. Seventeen NTDs (**Figure 1**) have been specified by the World Health Organization (WHO) and these include dengue, buruli ulcer, cutaneous leishmaniasis, taeniasis/cysticercosis and echinococcosis/hydatidosis, foodborne trematode infections, soil-transmitted helminthiasis (STH), intestinal worms, rabies, blinding trachoma, endemic treponematoses (yaws), leprosy, Chagas disease, Human African trypanosomiasis, visceral leishmaniasis, dracunculiasis, lymphatic filariasis, onchocerciasis and schistosomiasis [2]. These NTDs impair physical and intellectual capacities of the affected persons, thereby perpetuating the cycle of poverty [1]. Forty-seven countries in the African region are endemic to at least one NTD and 37 of them (79%) are coendemic for at least five of these diseases [3].

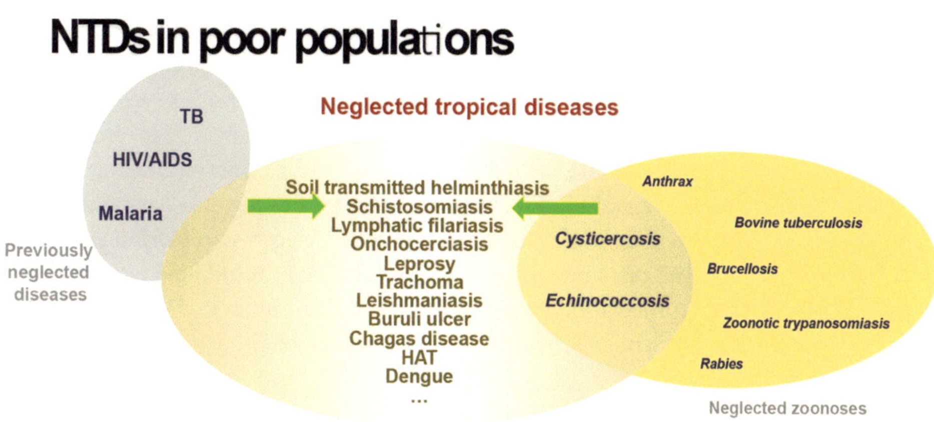

Figure 1. A list of neglected tropical diseases. Much attention is given to the previously neglected diseases being Malaria, HIV/AIDS and TB. While schistosomiasis and soil transmitted helminthiasis continue to be neglected. Included are neglected zoonosis diseases that come about the interactions of humans and their animals.

Five of the 17 NTDs [lymphatic filariasis, onchocerciasis, schistosomiasis, soil-transmitted helminthiasis (STH) and trachoma] are amenable to preventive chemotherapy. Thus, targeting such disease for control and elimination using available safe medicines and supported by complementary interventions could provide a noticeable quick win on NTD for the African region and in particular for the endemic countries. STHs have been specified as endemic in many countries even though the data collection methods used could be at variance from those recommended by WHO [3]. Countries in the African region through their Ministries of Health have not only endorsed the adoption of the resolutions on NTD by the World Health Assembly (WHA) in 2013, but they also expressed their commitment to scaling up interventions against the major NTDs [1]. With such an increased momentum to eliminate NTDs, it is critical that WHO member states implement NTD strategies demonstrating their commitments.

2. Disease transmission

Schistosomiasis transmission begins most often when people come into contact with bodies of freshwater in which infected people have urinated or defecated and there is a stage of the life cycle in intermediate snail host [4]. Transmission is linked to the life cycle of the schistosome (e.g., egg, miracidium larval form, sporocyst, cercaria, schistosomule, adult schistosome), when an egg comes in contact with freshwater, where it hatches and releases a miracidium. The miracidium swims by ciliary movement toward the snail intermediate host and penetrates its soft tissue. The *Schistosoma* species are transmitted by different freshwater snails that serve as intermediate hosts (**Figure 2**). The miracidium penetrated the snail and develops into sporocyst that migrates to the hepatic and gonadal tissue of the intermediate snail host. After 2–4 weeks, the sporocysts develop into cercariae [4]. Hundreds of the fork-tailed cercariae leave the snail intermediate host under the stimulation of light, swimming in the water until they find definitive mammalian hosts. The cercariae enters the skin using both mechanical activity and proteolytic enzymes [5], losing the tail and develops into schistosomules that migrate via the blood or lymphatic vessels [4]. The schistosomules then migrate to the portal circulation where they mature into adult worms. Adult *S. japonicum, S. mekongi* and *S. intercalatum* worms stay in the portal and mesenteric vessels, while *S. haematobium* worms migrate and live in the vesical plexus. The adult worms mate, with the male adult schistosome embracing the female worm into its gynaecophoric canal [5]. Four to 6 weeks after the cercaria has penetrated the human skin, the embraced female adult worm starts producing eggs, except for *S. haematobium* worms that take about 60–63 days before oviposition [6]. The adult female worms continue producing eggs throughout their lifetime, with about half the number of eggs produced are excreted with feces or urine, while the rest remain trapped in the tissues causing immunopathology (**Figure 2**) [7].

2.1. Global public health significance of schistosomiasis

Schistosomiasis remains one of the most prevalent parasitic diseases in the world, found endemic in 76 countries and is a public health concern in the developing world [8]. Schistoso-

http://dx.doi.org/10.5772/65282

miasis is a chronic disease, poorly recognized at early stages and if untreated the disease debilitates men and women during their most reproductive years. The disease is typically common in areas of the economically disadvantaged people living in areas that have no access to proper sanitation and good water supply systems. The high-risk groups for schistosomiasis are school age children, adolescents, reproductive women and also those whose occupations involve contact with water, for example fishermen, farmers, irrigation workers and women in their domestic tasks [8]. It is estimated that about 652 million people are at risk of infection from the five human schistosome species (*S. haematobium, S. mansoni, S. japonicum, S. intercalatum and S. mekongi*) and that 193 million are infected of which 85% are on the African continent [8]. Children between 5 and 15 years of age are the high-risk group and suffer most from morbidity due to high intensities of infection [9]. Though schistosomiasis has been intensively investigated over the past half a century, alone or in combination with other infectious diseases, a lot needs to be understood. **Figure 3** gives a detailed analysis of the effects of infection, the clinical evolution and the resultant severe diseases resolution and manifestations. Progression to disease severity is compounded by many other conditions that include the host genetics, coinfections by other parasites, intensity and duration of infection. However, other conditions such as malnutritional status of the host that is common in resource-limited areas may also aggravate the infections to severe diseases condition.

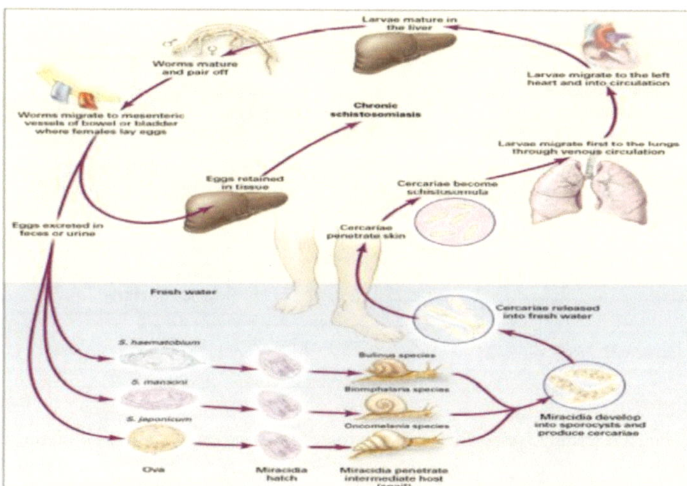

Figure 2. A general life cycle of *schistosome* species [7]. The life cycle shows the different shell morphology of the intermediate host and the morphological appearance of the ova that is important for diagnosis.

The number of individuals with hydronephrosis due to *S. haematobium* infection has been estimated to be close to 20 million, while about 70 million mainly school–age children suffer from hematuria due to their water contact activities [8]. Indirect measurement of morbidity is important in children, ranging from malnutrition, anemia, growth retardation, irritability and cognitive impairment that result in poor performance in school. Sick children are often absent from school, leading to loss in school performance and participation. Chronic irreversible sequelae, such as liver fibrosis, urinary tract obstruction and bladder cancer, become apparent in schistosomiasis in adult age as a result of heavy infection that occurs during childhood. This underscores the importance of repeated chemotherapy at regular intervals of young children living in endemic areas in order to prevent development of irreversible sequelae in adulthood.

Genital schistosomiasis is also common in both males and females in endemic areas. Female genital schistosomiasis (FGS) described as the presence of schistosome eggs on the upper or lower part of the reproductive tract has been demonstrated in up to 75% of females living in schistosomiasis endemic communities (**Figure 4A** and **B**) in Africa [10–12]. Reproductive complications due to FGS include low birthweight, abortions, ectopic pregnancies, primary and secondary infertility [13–16]. In African cultures, infertility in married couples is often blamed on women. This leads to rejection by husbands, family and kinship group. The society may not accept women who do not get pregnant [16]. It is also hypothesized that FGS facilitates transmission of HIV [12, 17]. The far-reaching consequences of schistosomiasis infection also include reduced national economic growth and persistent poverty. However, treatment using a single dose is now available, effective and safe to be taken by uninfected children or pregnant mothers and, can easily be incorporated into regular field activities [18]. Any initiative to control schistosomiasis will not only contribute towards morbidity reduction but also to the control of HIV transmission, improvement of school health and performance of children, national economic growth and poverty alleviation.

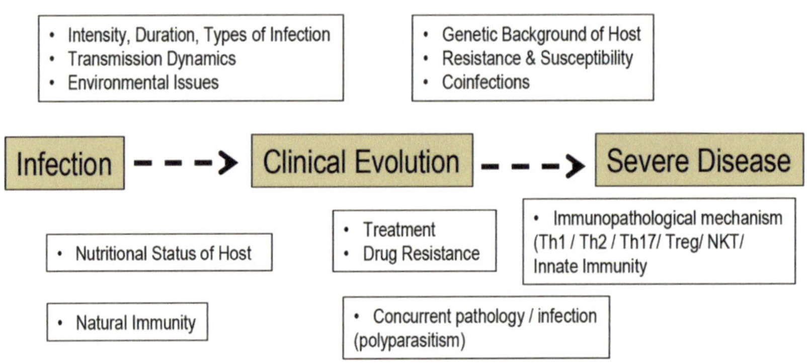

Figure 3. Indicating the contributing factors that drive one parasitic infection to clinical evolution and ultimately leading to severe diseases.

2.2. Soil-transmitted helminthiasis

Soil-transmitted helminthiases are nematodes transmitted from the soil to humans. These include hookworms (*Ancylostoms*), round worms (Ascaris *lumbricoides*) and whip worms (*Trichuris trichiura*). Like schistosomiasis, soil transmitted helminthes (STHs) are widely distributed in economically disadvantaged communities who do not have sanitary facilities [19]. The burden of the disease associated with STHs is enormous. Over two billion people are infected worldwide and 135,000 people die annually from STHs infection [2, 19]. Again like schistosomiasis, the most susceptible groups are primary and preschool-aged children (5–15 years). About 400 million school age children worldwide are infected with STHs [3]. Hookworm infection is picked at the age of two years when children are frequently left to play on contaminated soil and infection increases with age, age range (5–15 years) being the most high-risk group [19, 20]. Hookworm infection causes iron-deficient anemia [21]. The intestinal stage hookworms feed on blood and cause further hemorrhage when they stop feeding because they release anticoagulant compounds. A single adult hookworm is estimated to cause a daily blood loss into the gut of from 0.03 to 0.15 ml [21, 22]. Intestinal stage hookworms change position every 4–6 h as they seek new sites for blood meal [23]. This mode of feeding is a major cause of morbidity in young children and pregnant women who have high demand of iron or are malnourished. Other effects of hookworm infection include itchy rash, cough, fever, bloody sputum, and loss of appetite, nausea, vomiting, diarrhea, abdominal discomfort, paleness, fatigue and blood in the stool [21].

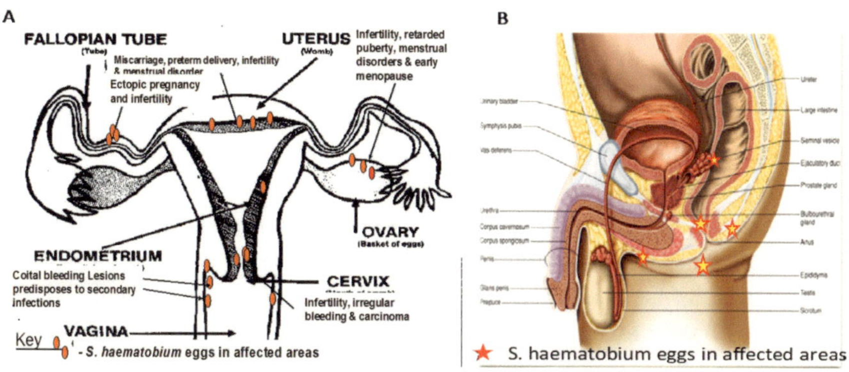

Figure 4. Illustration of the female (A) and male (B) genital schistosomiasis affected areas. The affected areas may facilitate easy transmission of HIV besides causing other reproductive complication leading to infertility.

Ascaris lumbricoides infection causes diarrhea, intestinal obstruction, reduced food intake, abdominal pains, impaired fat digestion and Vitamin A absorption (leading to nutritional deficiency). Infected children contaminate the soil by their indiscriminate defecation. Infection causes reduced appetite leading to malnutrition, which in turn result in reduced host immune resistance to other infections. Other effects include vomiting, jaundice, disturbed sleep, dry skin and pneumonitis during larval passage in lungs. *Trichuris trichiura* (whipworm) cause blood loss in the form of hemorrhage associated with trichuriasis dysentery syndrome or rectal prolapse [22]. More commonly blood loss is believed to be part of an exudation from the damaged epithelium and is proportional to parasite burden. Other effects of whipworm infection include: diarrhea and pain in the right lower abdomen, anemia secondary to blood loss and impaired learning (cognitive) ability [23]. Transmission of *Ascaris lumbricoides* and *Trichuris trichiura* is through oral fecal route by ingestion of infective eggs. Children who are most frequently exposed to contaminated soils are mostly infected than adults.

The conditions that support transmission of STH are similar to those favoring transmission of schistosomiasis (poor sanitation, contamination of the environment with human excreta, poverty leading to lack of protective clothing and safe water supply). These conditions could create an overlap of epidemiological distribution of schistosomiasis and STHs in some regions. There is a high risk of morbidity exacerbation due to mixed infection from schistosomes and STHs. At least 50% of severely ill people due to worm infestation are school age children [19, 24], and infection from STHs and schistosomiasis represent more than 40% of the disease burden due to all tropical diseases, excluding malaria [25]. But these diseases are treatable. The public health significance of schistosomiasis and STH has triggered response from WHO, which in the 54.19th WHA 2001, demanded that all member state endemic to these NTDs should provide regular mass treatment to primary school children at risk of morbidity due to schistosomiasis and STH, with praziquantel and albendazole. There is a major shift in the policy for the control of Preventative Chemotherapeutic Treatment of NTDs to that of control/elimination [3].

2.3. Diagnosis

The standard diagnosis for schistosomiasis is detection of viable eggs in urine (*S. haematobium*), feces (*S. japonicum, S. mansoni*), or tissue biopsies. Currently, the presence of infecting schistosomes cannot be ruled out definitively if no ova are detected in urine or feces, because of the low sensitivity of the standard urine and fecal examinations [26]. Molecular techniques to detect schistosome DNA in fecal specimens have greater sensitivity than microscopy, but the techniques still suffer from sampling limitations because of the irregular distribution of eggs in the excreta. Schistosome DNA detection in serum or urine is being evaluated [27]. Serological assays have proven useful for diagnosis as the techniques detect schistosome-antigen–specific antibodies in symptomatic individuals. However, for individuals in endemic areas for schistosomiasis, the serology is unable to discriminate between active infection and past exposure. The main challenge of the serological assays is the inability to distinguish between past and current active infection. However, a negative test can rule out infection in endemic population, while another drawback is the test positivity over prolonged periods after therapy making the tests unreliable for post-treatment follow-up [27]. Better diagnostic tests for schistosomiasis are still needed for both in the field and in the clinic and new technologies are being studied. Advances for drug development is also essential for diseases elimination programs and vaccine assessment in which infection follow-up post-treatment must be accurately monitored over time. Currently, there is a lack of true gold standard for quantitative correlations to the actual worm burden [26]. An important public health aspect of monitoring control and elimination programs would be detection of schistosome infections in the snail host. Snail xenodiagnosis would enable the identification of environmental contamination especially during the control and elimination programs by the use of snails located at selected sentinel sites or assessing wild snails at common water contact sites [27]. The snail infections are usually detected by inducing cercarial shedding, while prepatent infections can be identified using histological examination of snail tissues and molecular parasitological techniques such as polymerase chain reaction (PCR) or loop-mediated isothermal amplification assays [28].

2.4. Global control of helminthiasis

2.4.1. Vector control

The three major species of schistosomes that infect humans, *S. mansoni, S. haematobium* and *S. japonicum,* are transmitted by specific genera of snails; *Biomphalaria spp., Bulinus spp.* and *Oncomelania spp.,* respectively. Vector control has most commonly been done through the use of chemical molluscicides such as niclosamide [29]. The chemicals that kill snails are nonspecific and are also toxic for other aquatic life such as fish. Fish toxicity and yellowing of treated water by niclosamide decrease the acceptability of mollusciciding by the communities [30]. The chemicals are expensive, while they can rapidly be washed down streams following rains or diluted to nontoxic concentrations in larger water bodies, thereby demanding frequent reapplication. Furthermore, training for personnel who apply molluscicides is required who would understand the environmental conditions such as water hardness and temperature.

Indigenous plant extracts are an attractive alternative to chemicals for killing snails. These have low costs due to local availability and the extracts are less toxic to other forms of aquatic life [31]. The plant *Phytolacca dodecandra* has received some attention but has not been effectively employed for schistosomiasis control. The intervention requires community involvement that is dependent on participation rates that is affected by perceived importance of the intervention, the ability to observe impact or personal benefits and the degree of input the population has in designing the intervention [32]. Biological control is another approach to reducing snail populations and impacting transmission of schistosomiasis. Prawns and crawfish can be used to reduce snail populations, for example, *M. vollenhovenii* and *Procambarus clarkii* are voracious consumers of snails. Certain species of fish are also predators for the snails that transmit schistosomiasis. Cichlid populations are molluscivores that preferentially feed on *Bulinus spp.* compared to snails with thicker shells [33]. Other attempts to alter snail populations include environmental alterations such as removal of vegetation on which they feed, lining canals with cement or draining water bodies where they live [34]. Attempts to directly remove snails that included financial incentives for numbers of snails collected have been employed but with increased infection risk to persons doing the work [35]. The applicability and efficacy of this method in African settings is not appropriate. While in areas of high schistosomiasis transmission, it has been reported that the number of infected snails is usually low, suggesting that only a few infected snails maintain the life cycle [36]. Snails that are nonhosts for human schistosomiasis and compete with or predate on intermediate host snails can be used for control. Introduction of ampullarid (e.g., *Marisa cornuarietis*) or thiarid (e.g., *Melanoides tuberculata*) snails in endemic areas in the Caribbean region was reported to successfully displace populations of *Biomphalaria spp.* leading to reduction and interruption of *S. mansoni* of transmission [37].

2.4.2. Health education

Health education is an important component of effective schistosomiasis prevention and control. Developing health education programs requires that the design, administration and outcomes be adapted to different socioeconomic and cultural settings [38]. Several studies have shown that the individual's behavioral changes facilitating disease prevention and control. Behavior cannot be changed simply with the acquisition of knowledge that can be obtained from health education [39]. Health education programs end up not successful when the socioeconomic and cultural context of communities is not considered. Individuals and communities have to be considered in full their environment and education when developing programs for the control of diseases in an area. The success of programs in reducing high-risk behavior and promoting health-enhancing behavior depends to a considerable degree on whether the life cycle and other biomedical concepts and information are presented in an appropriate, emotional, social, economic and cultural context of target populations. Consideration should be taken when people do not have the means for changing their behavior, for example, inadequate health services, no access to proper sanitation and clean water supply, unavailability of antihelminthic medications and unaffordability of modern treatment.

Observations were made in a longitudinal study conducted in Zimbabwe over 33 months in which parasitology follow-up examination and treatment was done every 6 months for the first year, then a break for almost 24 months. The reinfection was observed to take place in such an endemic setting rising to almost half the levels before treatment (**Figures 5A–D**). However, after a long break of 24 months, the prevalence was seen to rise to almost pretreatment levels, even though infection intensity was drastically reduced.

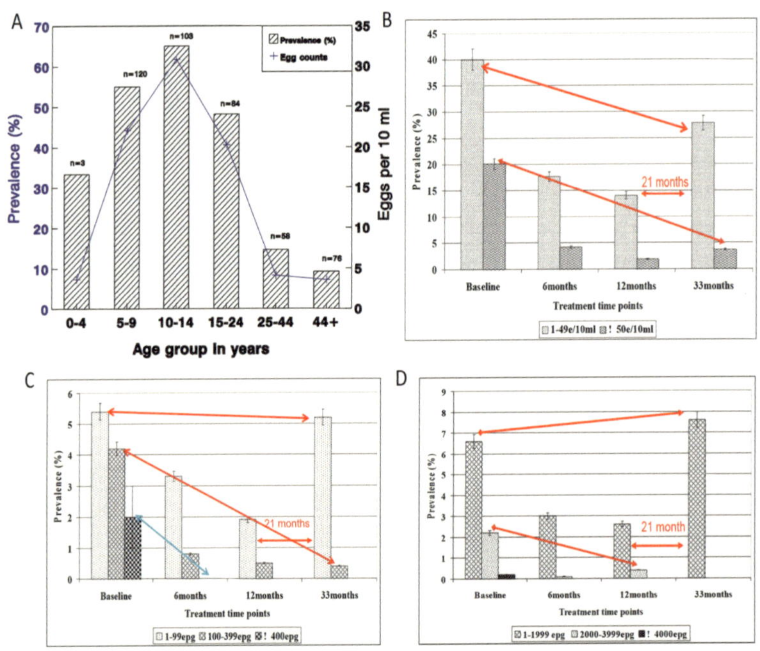

Figure 5. Showing a typical infection re-infection longitudinal study conducted in Zimbabwe at 6 monthly observations in the first year and then another examination after 24 months. **Panel A**: A typical age prevalence/egg intensity curve in a community before treatment. Showing a peak within the 10–14-year-old age group. **Panel B**: *S. haematobium;* **Panel C**: *S. mansoni* and **Panel D**: Soil-transmitted helminths; infection prevalence and intensity of infection with follow-up time point. Regular treatment was observed to be effective in prevention of heavy infections.

2.4.3. *Vaccines*

Despite several years of mass antiparasitic drug therapy programs and other control measures, helminthiasis still continues to exist. The discovery of a vaccine still remains a pipe dream for the control of human helminthiasis. A vaccine would contribute to the reduction of schistosomiasis morbidity through immune modulation leading to a decrease in parasite load and reduced egg production. A lot of research has been done with a view of controlling and preventing schistosomiasis. Researchers have focused on vaccines, host genetic predisposition, coinfections, autoimmunity and improved diagnostics for surveillance.

Several candidate human schistosomiasis vaccines are in different stages of preclinical and clinical development. The most eligible candidates are egg antigens and the schistosomula tegument membrane antigens (Sm 23, SmTSP-2 and Sm29) [40] of *S. haematobium* and *S. mansoni*. Two recombinant *S. mansoni* vaccines; *Sm*-TSP-2 and *Sm*-14 are being tested, while *Sm*p80 (calpain) is undergoing testing in nonhuman primates [40]. The *Sh*28GST, also known as Bilhvax is in advanced clinical development for *S. haematobium* infection. These vaccines were selected on the basis of their protective immunity in preclinical challenge models, through human immune-epidemiological studies or both [41]. The vaccine candidate development and evaluations are being advanced through collaboration of academic research institutions, nonprofit vaccine product development partnerships, biotechnology companies, and developing country vaccine manufacturers. The success in developing promising vaccine candidates has been possible from screening schistosome *OMICs* databases using DNA microarray profiling, proteomics, glycomics and immunomics [42] and the application of RNA interference (RNAi) technology that has allowed investigators to ascribe specific functions to the parasite molecules and the role in parasite survival [43]. A potential strategy that could accelerate the achievement of an effective vaccine would be the association of different recombinant antigens that previously resulted in partial protection or the use of pools of antigens known as multivalent or multiepitope vaccines [42].

The vaccine development strategies are bedeviled with many biological bottlenecks such as the lack of reliable surrogates of protection in humans; immune interactions in coinfections with other diseases in endemic areas; the potential risk of IgE responses to antigens in endemic populations; and paucity of appropriate vaccine efficacy studies in nonhuman primate models. Research is also needed on the role of modern adjuvants targeting specific parts of the innate immune system to tailor a potent and protective immune response for lead schistosome vaccine candidates with the long-term aim to achieve curative worm reduction [44].

3. Immunology

Immune responses during schistosomiasis can be considered in terms of three broad aspects of immunopathogenesis, resistance to reinfection and immunodiagnostics. The development and establishment of chronic infection is impacted by the presence of chronic antigenic exposure as illustrated in **Figure 2** and summarized in **Figure 3**. The immunological regulation associated with the morbidity of schistosomiasis has been studied without completely understanding the impact [45, 46] of the immunological components involved that contribute to failure to design successful vaccines. However, the immune mechanisms related to resistance to reinfection and in response to candidate parasite antigens are not well defined. Adult worms are known to be refractory to immune attack; while immature and developing worms, skin-stage and lung-stage schistosomulae are the probable targets of protective immunity [46, 47] that are safe from drug effects. Whether a protective resistance to reinfection exists is still not well characterized and understood [47, 48], but evidence suggests that such resistance may develop rather slowly [46, 47]. The induction of protective immunity has been shown through immunization of various experimental hosts with irradiated cercariae to work for a short period of time. Data from endemic populations suggest that age-associated decreases in infection result from the development of antiparasite immunity, rather than reduced contact with water [24]. Although the responsible antigens and host immune responses are not fully defined, resistance to reinfection is believed to be associated with IgE antibodies against worm antigens, with low concentrations of IgG4 antibodies to worm antigens and high blood eosinophilia. Resistance to reinfection is partial, which means that protective sterile immunity either does not develop or is rare. Treatment of schistosomiasis increases common correlates of resistance: eosinophilia, parasite-specific IgE and interleukin 5 production in response to worm antigens, while repeated treatment to prevent reinfections can lead to longer intervals before reinfection, even accounting for similar exposure patterns in highly exposed participants [48].

3.1. Coinfections

Neglected tropical diseases are found in areas that have conducive environmental conditions. Schistosomiasis and soil-transmitted helminthiasis often occur alongside each other and with other tropical infectious diseases and with a wide range of coinfecting organisms. In addition to the direct morbidities, schistosomiasis can affect immunological and physiological responses of the host and the coinfecting pathogens. Thus, better control of schistosomiasis could provide adjunctive benefits towards other coinfecting organisms in such areas. The most studied and compelling example is the effect of schistosomiasis on susceptibility to HIV infection. Among women with female genital schistosomiasis, the inflammation of the genital epithelial tissue can lead to a compromised physical barrier to exposure to HIV through sexual activity. In population-based studies, female genital schistosomiasis has been associated with a three to four times increased risk of HIV infection [10–12, 16, 17, 49].

Schistosomiasis alters immune responses directed towards coinfecting pathogens, allergens or vaccines. The immunoregulatory responses during schistosome infection could downregulate T-helper type-1 immune response associated with the control of viral or protozoan infections or interfere with immunization generally made available to children living in affected tropical areas. In one of many studies of schistosomiasis and malaria coinfections it seems to indicate that schistosomiasis modulates malaria; however, studies have yielded conflicting results [50–54]. In some cases, malaria prevalence, anemia and pathological effects are higher in children with schistosomiasis than in children without schistosomiasis, whereas antimalarial immune responses are diminished [51]. However, other studies report no protective effect of schistosome infection on malaria that can be accompanied by increased immune responses [53, 54]. Schistosome and malaria-related antigens can cross react to some extent, further complicating the situation. However, within the host there is need for a delicate but subtle interplay between pro- and anti-inflammatory cytokines that play a major controlling effector role on the antibody production and the cell-mediated antibody dependent cytotoxicity (**Figure 6A** and **B**).

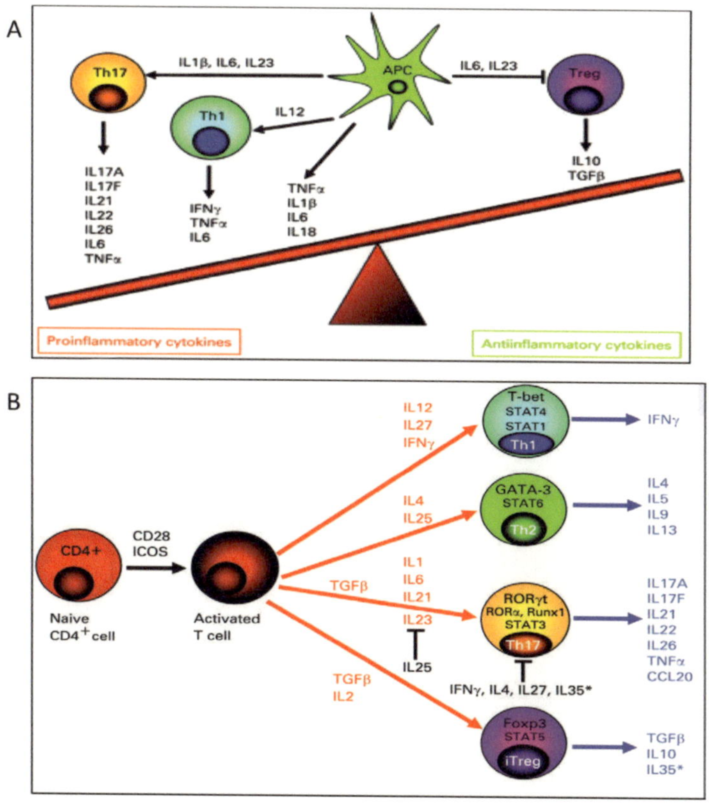

Figure 6. Plate A, Pro- and anti-inflammatory cytokines involved in a delicate balances that play an important role in down regulating deleterious effector response to helminthiasis invasion. **Plate B**, Illustrating the key T-helper subsets that are important in helminthiasis infections, control and regulation to avoid development of immunopathology.

3.2. Host immunogenetics

The development of genetic epidemiology methods using recent human genetic mapping information has led to major advances in the identification of host genes in human schistosomiasis and other infections [55]. Determining the role of host genetics in schistosomiasis is complicated by the numerous parasite and environmental factors involved in transmission. Two immunological and pathological phenotypes have been studied so far as schistosomiasis infection levels on the host-parasite as consequences measured by the fecal egg counts and the severe hepatic fibrosis assessed by ultrasound examination. The first study was performed on

Brazilian pedigrees and provided strong evidence for a major gene controlling infection levels by *S. mansoni* denoted as SM1, which was mapped to chromosome 5q31-q33 [55]. This region contains several candidate genes involved in the regulation of the Th1/Th2 responses. The direct role of cytokine polymorphisms located within these genes further elucidation. Another study conducted in Sudan showed the presence of a major gene influencing the development of severe hepatic fibrosis during *S. mansoni* infection denoted as SM2. This gene is located on chromosome 6q22-q23 and is closely linked to the IFN-gamma receptor 1 gene encoding the receptor of the strongly antifibrogenic cytokine interferon-gamma. There is also evidence for the genetic control of pathology due to *S. mansoni*, where the linkage is reported on a region containing the gene for the interferon-gamma receptor 1 subunit. Numerous association studies have also provided evidence for major histocompatibility complex control of pathology in schistosomiasis through cytokine polymorphisms [55–57]. Host immunogenetics is important in driving the host immune effector mechanisms such that cytokine polymorphisms may be crucial in the expression of resistance or susceptibility to a host of infections [57, 58]. Any impact on the underlying immune genetics (**Figure 7**), would impact the cytokines expression and antibody production [58].

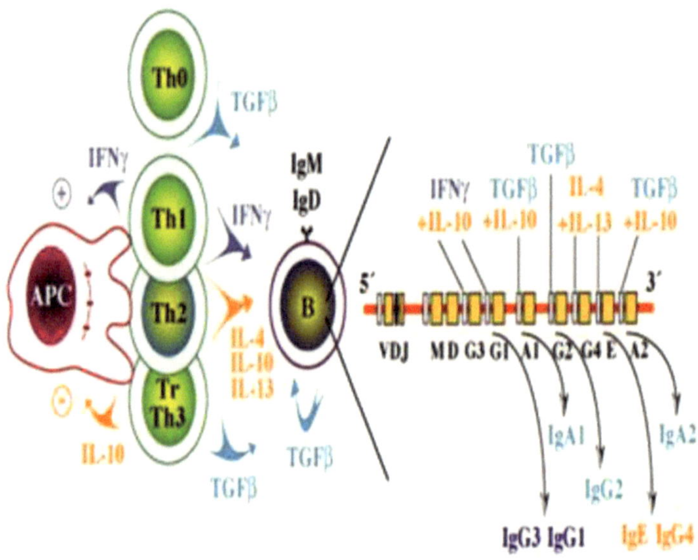

Figure 7. Showing the link of the antigen presentation to the T-helper cell subsets including T-regulatory cells. The T-helper cells produce a barrage of cytokines that selectively influence B cells at gene level to class switch antibody production leading to the synthesis of either protective or blocking antibodies [58].

4. Mass drug administration (MDA)

Mass drug administrations (MDA) in affected populations or communities form the basis of current schistosomiasis and soil-transmitted helminthiasis (STH) control and/or management.

The MDAs can follow one or more of the following approaches; house-to-house administrations (i.e., mobile teams), booth distribution (i.e., fixed teams), administering drugs in special population groups (e.g., school age children, etc.) and/or areas of community gatherings (e.g., marketplaces, stations, etc.) [2]. Such chemotherapeutic prevention and management strategies of infectious diseases in endemic areas have some significant shortcomings, chief among them being re-infections [59, 60], due to untreated human and animal reservoirs. Prophylactic measures in these areas are difficult as that would mean people will have to take the medicines frequently for life, thus exposing them to potential life-threatening adverse drug events and development of drug resistance. In endemic areas during a five-year round of annual mass treatment of school going age children, before and post-treatment checks revealed that re-infection always takes place (**Figure 5**). Reinfections were most common in cases where MDA was not accompanied with adequate environmental and health promotion/education interventions. Successful MDA in endemic areas has to be conducted in all age groups. For better coverage, the World Health Organization recommends the utilization of all available medicine distribution channels especially in countries with high levels of infections [60–64].

Repeated MDAs have helped some countries to significantly reduce the disease burden. An example is the 84% reduction of baseline levels of schistosomiasis in a moderately highly endemic region of the northeast of Sierra Leone, with MDA interventions repeated yearly over three years [61]. Communities in Zanzibar, Tanzania also recorded significant reductions in infections levels of soil-transmitted helminthiasis (90–98%) and scabies (68–98%) as additional benefits associated with the annual mass drug administration of ivermectin and albendazole for lymphatic filariasis. Modeling done by Anderson *et al.* [62] noted that it was possible to even eliminate *S. mansoni* by WHO's MDA guidelines at least in areas with lower transmission levels if high coverage is attained and maintained beyond above 75% coverage [64]. The noted disease burden reductions also have positive impact on morbidities and comorbidities like anemia, malaria and HIV [49, 64].

Despite significant contributions, great optimism and positive outlook; MDA may not lead to total elimination on its own [63]. There is a great need for critical assessments of all MDAs for more positive effects to be realized. Significant community effectiveness of MDA programs stand challenged by issues around; very low coverage (<75%) as about a third of those that really require treatment and/or chemoprophylaxis are receiving it [64, 65]; the utilization of volunteers and/or underpaid workers to distribute or administer medicines; overly relying on fragile healthcare systems in marginalized communities or countries; lack of health and/or pharmacoeconomic evaluations; sustainability questions associated with all chemo-prophylaxis interventions; belief systems, socioeconomic status and general community acceptance; lack of evidence of wider safety and effectiveness of medicines involved in different communities and fears of exerting unnecessary selection pressure, thus promoting drug resistance [63–65]. Despite the noted negative concerns, MDA remain popular in the prevention and/or management of schistosomiasis and soil transmitted helminthiasis. As highlighted above WHO suggests ways by which wider coverage can be attained like utilization of all available medicine distribution channels. Also because in almost all affected and/or poor countries developmental partners and international pharmaceutical companies finance the MDAs, as such the programs remain cost-effective at least from a governmental perspective of pharmacoeconomic evaluations. Issues to do with community acceptance may be addressed by adequate promotional and/or educational programs to clearly explain the aims and objectives of each MDA intervention. Critical evaluation of each MDA intervention on issues to do with safety, drug effectiveness, cost-effectiveness/benefit, sustainability and political will positively feed into the subsequent interventions.

4.1. Helminthiasis management

For schistosomiasis, WHO recommends praziquantel with doses of 40–60 mg/kg body weight in one and/or 2–3 divided dose(s). Praziquantel is effective against all five important species of schistosomes, that is, *Schistosoma mansoni, S. haematobium, S. japonicum, S. intercalatum* and *S. mekongi*. Praziquantel 'the first antihelminthic drug to fulfill the World Health Organization's requirements for population-based chemotherapy of a broad range of parasitic infections' is also effective against clonorchiasis, opisthorchiasis, paragonimiasis, taeniasis and intestinal trematodiases. Other drugs with recognizable effectiveness against schistosomiasis are metrifonate and oxamniquine. Metrifonate is an organophosphate cholinesterase inhibitor thus it has significant safety issues. Oxamniquine has a complicated manufacturing process, which drives manufacturing cost up [65]. Thus, oxamniquine costs way more than praziquantel, making it unfavorable for wider mass usage. Praziquantel was demonstrated to be way more effective as compared to oxamniquine, when used in a controlled trial cure rate for praziquantel was high (96.1%) while that of oxamniquine was low (42.4%) [66]. Praziquantel remains the first and only choice in all cases of schistosomiasis owing to its low cost, high efficacy, low toxicity and ease of administration. The acceptable attribute is mostly single oral doses that enhances compliance.

The mechanism of action of praziquantel is thought to involve the increased permeability to Ca^{2+} ions leading to uncontrollable contractions, paralysis and death of the worm. It is also suggested that it leads to vacuolation and blebbing of worm tegumental and subtegumental structures in adults but not juveniles worms [67, 68]. This leads to the exposure of surface antigens to host immune system thus Facilitating immune recognition and clearance of the worm [67]. The drug effect may be explained due to relative differences in sensitivities observed in some settings between adult and juvenile worms [67]. Praziquantel is well absorbed orally (80%), is subjected to first pass effect, metabolized by the liver and excreted via the kidneys [19]. Microsomal enzymes inducers like rifampicin interfere negatively with praziquantel efficacy as they lead to lower than minimum effective concentration of praziquantel in the blood. On the other hand, CYP450 inhibitors like cimetidine, ketoconazole, grape juice, etc. may lead to higher than normal blood levels. It is contraindicated in patients with history of epilepsy and those hypersensitive to it. Operation of machinery or driving by individual after intake is not recommended. There is no evidence linking praziquantel to mutagenesis or harmful effects to fetuses. But as a general rule drugs are best avoided in the first trimester and used during the rest of pregnancy when benefits outweighs risks [19]. The usual mild side effects of praziquantel which generally do not require treatment are malaise, headache, dizziness, abdominal discomfort with or without nausea and/or vomiting, fever and urticarial. Some of these side effects may be altogether the effects of schistosomiasis. These and other side effects may be worse in patients with high worm burden. Resistance to praziquantel by schistosomes has not been reported as yet, as there are no substantiated clinical findings. Reports of resistance are usually misrepresentations of issues like noncompliance or very transient biological phenomena or effects [67, 68].

4.1.1. Management of soil-transmitted helminthiasis

In the management of STH, the WHO recommends any of the following drugs: albendazole (dose of 400 mg); mebendazole (dose of 500 mg); levamisole (dose of 2.5 $mgkg^{-1}$) and pyrantel (dose of 10 $mgkg^{-1}$). These drugs are effective against many helminthic infections, for example ascariasis, hookworms, lymphatic filariasis, trichuriasis, strongyloidiasis, zoonotic ancylostomiasis, enterobiasis, among others. Benzimidazoles (i.e., albendazole and mebendazole) are the mostly commonly used [58, 65] in the management of STHs owing to their efficacy, wider spectrum, safety and availability. Benzimidazoles are thought work through inhibiting tubulin polymerisation. Absorption of albendazole is usually very low and the absorbed is subjected to significant first pass effect by the liver. Mebendazole is absorbed almost fourfold better than albendazole, but the rest are similar. May cause bone marrow suppression if taken for a considerable long period as in hydatid disease management were the patient takes three 28 day cycles with 14 day breaks of albendazole. Benzimidazoles are best avoided in pregnancy especially during the first trimester unless good clinical advice benefits outweigh risks [19]. Without having the pharmacokinetic properties changed, praziquantel increases plasma concentration and area under the curve of albendazole sulfoxide (the most active metabolite) by about 50% in healthy subjects. This might be beneficial in coadministration as in MDAs, but also may lead to more side/adverse effects. Side/adverse effects of albendazole depending on the duration of therapy may include, abdominal pain, nausea and vomiting, fever, elevated hepatic enzymes, dizziness, headache, meningeal signs, raised intracranial pressure and vertigo hypersensitivity

Benzimidazoles are active against *Ascaris lumbricoides, Enterobius vermicularis, Necator americanus, Ancylostoma duodenale,* Trichuriasis, Strongyloidiasis, *Trichinella spiralis,* neurocysticercosis, cystic hydatid disease and microspiridiosis. Resistance to albendazole though rare occurs through alteration of the target site. The other drugs highlighted above are better reserved for drug-resistant worms. Levamisole is now in most guidelines reserved for veterinary use. Also, pyrantel has an inferior effective profile as compared to benzimidazoles. For long-term solutions, there is a need to combine MDA with various other strategies like improving the quality of the water supply, sanitation and hygiene, education and health promotion and intensify the search for vaccine development. Levamisole and pyrantel are not widely used, but since they are not in the same class as albendazole and mebendazole, they are usually reserved for drug-resistant forms of STHs. Thus, MDAs with praziquantel and a benzimidazole have a wide spectrum covering against important helminths. Coadministration has additional benefits that can be realized if regular MDAs are done in affected communities.

4.1.2. Safety of combining praziquantel and benzimidazoles

High safety profile has been observed, in a safety study of praziquantel – albendazole combined treatment of hydatidosis, which require a way more prolonged duration than schistosomiasis and/or STHs [69]. The mild side effects noted were not so different from when monotherapies were used and were transient, disappearing when treatment was withdrawn [69]. There may be need for more evaluations of the severity of side and/or adverse-effects versus worm burden, when worms are localized in the central nervous system and/or in eyes.

4.2. New chemotherapeutic avenues

Mathematical models suggest significant drug resistance by the helminths to current therapies in the new future [70], the need for new, safer and more effective drugs is apparent. It has been demonstrated that the use of praziquantel and other drugs may enhance the antischistosomal activity. An example of such drugs is lovastatin [65] (a hypolipidemic agent). Benzodiazepines such as clonazepam are known to have the ability to paralyze adult schistosomes (both males and females) and interfere with egg release [65]. Other promising molecules with antischistosomal activities are the artemisinins and related 1,2,4-trioxolanes [68]. Praziquantel and artemisinin derivatives combined offers better protection [69] and/or cure rates. Though not 100% effective, MDAs based on WHO guidelines are very important in the fight against many parasitic neglected tropical diseases like schistosomiasis and soil transmitted helminthiasis. MDAs has actually more benefits due to the wider spectrum of both praziquantel and albendazole/mebendazole, as the administration will cover other parasitic infections within targeted communities. Effectiveness is significantly improved if chemoprophylaxis is done together with education and promotion of hygiene and the use of safe water. While praziquantel and albendazole/mebendazole are very effective there is still need to develop new better pharmaceuticals and pursue other avenues like vaccines.

4.3. Schistosomiasis control and elimination: research priorities and capacity building needs

The WHO/TDR Special Program for Research and Training in Tropical Diseases convened diseases reference groups to examine and set research priorities for the neglected tropical diseases. The following research priorities were made: (i) to optimize existing intervention tools so as to maximize impact and sustainability, (ii) to develop novel control tools that will improve impact and sustainability, (iii) to improve diagnostic tests with good sensitivity, specificity, multiplex capacity, and ability to measure infection intensity, and detect drug resistance; especially useful at the current preventive treatment control initiative in which reinfection would be very low. There is also need (iv) to standardize and validate methodologies and cost effective protocols for diagnosis in monitoring and evaluation settings, (v) to develop delivery strategies of multiple interventions to maximize sustainability of control program and integrated neglected tropical diseases control. Recommendation also included the need to develop strategies to increase awareness of ill-health processes, community participation, ownership and empowerment, as well as equity in access to preventive chemotherapeutic control interventions. The application of epidemiological models is required to help monitoring of intervention efficacy including drug resistance tracing. Further to develop new tools for parasite functional genomics in key species, this is believed to assist in vaccine development. A comprehensive research agenda need to be developed from basic sciences to emphasize implementation research and to ensure that control program could be implemented and evaluated based on rigorous scientific evidence. New tools, policies and strategies would lead to strengthened control programs that aim at disease elimination or eradication, where feasible.

4.4. Progress of schistosomiasis preventive chemotherapy in the African region: challenges and research needs

The African region has the highest burden of schistosomiasis, with 4 intermediate host species, endemic in 43 countries. According to WHO statistics at least 220 million people may have schistosomiasis infections. Ten sub-Saharan countries account for more than 70% of the global number of people requiring preventive chemotherapy for schistosomiasis. Prevalence of infection and morbidity are high in school-age children, but high prevalence has also been documented in children less than 5 years of age [71, 72]. The African region has adopted and recommends a comprehensive control strategy for schistosomiasis that includes preventive chemotherapy, health education, access clean water, sanitation and environmental control. These strategies, if implemented vigorously, would lead to the reduction of morbidity and possibly interruption of transmission. However treatment coverage is low in the region and many countries are not yet mapped. Scaling up to reach at least 75% of children is still a challenge because of access to praziquantel. Treatment of pre-school children is also limited by the lack of a pediatric formulation [52].

Research priorities for schistosomiasis control and elimination in endemic region include, better understanding of the epidemiology and surveillance of infections, implementation research, environmental and social ecology, better use of data and modeling and the basic biology of transmission and snail dynamics [73]. These priorities can only be met through widespread capacity strengthening and collaborative partnerships, transparent interactions between researchers and disease control program managers, learning from areas that have successfully controlled and have experience in research and control of schistosomiasis, for example, China, including intersectorial collaboration and technology transfer and political commitment and funding for disease control and research in each affected country. Conduct of the required research should also be done so as to increase capacity for advanced research as well as to improve disease control. Capacity strengthening should provide personnel able to address gaps from the laboratory to the field, and with skills to properly evaluate interventions, model likely progression and scenarios and quantify impacts of the control program. For schistosomiasis control and elimination, it will be important to rebuild capacity for malacology, which was not stressed when preventive chemotherapy was the main operational component. Other aspects to be strengthened are drug efficacy monitoring, and pharmacovigilance.

4.5. Monitoring and evaluation towards the elimination of schistosomiasis

Monitoring and evaluation (M&E) is a process that helps to improve performance and achieve planned targets. The goal should be to improve current and future management of outputs, outcomes and impact. The results of M&E should help control programs, governments and development partners assess the performance and progress towards schistosomiasis control and elimination. These processes should also document past and current interventions, as well as for planning future activities. Monitoring should be incorporated and implemented from the planning stage of a program as a periodic and recurring task. Documenting results, processes and experiences should steer decision-making and learning processes. Monitoring checks progress against plans. The data acquired through monitoring is used for evaluation.

Evaluations should help to draw conclusions about efficiency, effectiveness, impact, relevance and sustainability of the interventions. The process consolidates information and allows program managers to learn from each other's experiences, building on expertise and knowledge; generates reports that contribute to transparency and accountability of donated resources. Evaluation may reveal errors and offers alternative ways for improvements. Evaluation documentation provides means by which agencies consolidate and learn from their experiences making policy to guide control and monitoring activities. Evaluations also provide ways to assess the success of the program and the relationship between implementers, decision makers and beneficiaries. Evaluation results provide evidence for raising funds, influencing policy and tracking the success of the program. The assessments of activities depend to a large extent on the manner in which monitoring and evaluation is recommended. Assessment of performance is necessary to select indicators that permit rating of the targeted outputs and outcomes before the implementation of the project.

Parasitological indicators: This aspect using parasitology to determine number of people screened for infection, number of people positive, number of people requiring preventive chemotherapy, number of people treated and the positive numbers to be treated.

Malacological indicators: The indicators here show the number of areas that need survey, the number of areas that are high transmission, the number of areas that need molluscicides/snail control and the number of areas that have been treated/modified.

There should be indicators for other interventions such as health education, water supply and sanitation. Evaluation should inform whether planned tasks are completed or on-going. Quality control and effectiveness of all interventions should be assured.

5. Concluding remarks: mass drug administration for the control of helminthiasis

Tropical and subtropical areas have conducive environment for the flourishing of helminthiasis; these include appropriate temperature, wet and humid soils, abundant fresh flowing river waters and the human factor that continuously contaminates their environment and maintains the life cycle of the parasites. Vaccines are still a long way to be developed since we lack complete understanding of the host-parasite relationship. Host-parasite effects have been observed those leading into severe pathology, in some instances, during the parasite colonization. The effects of helminthiasis are so diverse affecting the health of the host resulting in poor cognitive in school children, affecting reproductive health in child-bearing age and reduced work output in economically engaged workforce. The current control strategy is by removing the infection using preventive chemotherapy, ultimately anticipating cutting the life cycle of helminthiasis after several rounds of treatment using mass drug administration. While controlling the life cycle by treatment, much effort should be invested in health education to reduce contamination of the environment. The overall control strategies required should include health education, water and sanitation development, selective chemotherapy, snail control and passive treatment of cases. The options for consideration of water and sanitation development remain a major challenge since this is grossly neglected in most developing areas that are resource limited. While additional environmental and engineering measures for irrigation schemes particularly the small scale irrigation currently being developed require incorporation of the helminthiasis control strategy right from the onset of program development. Use of indigenous and locally available resources in vector control should be included in health education and basic health delivery services (e.g., plant molluscicide — *Phytolacca dodecandra)*. This can be grown as homestead or garden hedge whose berries can be crushed for local application at water contact sites for the control of snail vectors. Concerted efforts from all partners in human development need to be involved in the control of helminthiasis. Partnerships with other sectors in the farming, irrigation, health education and mining is required for the common goal to develop and improve human living standards in an effort to control helminthiasis from all angles.

Finally, recommendations are made for comprehensive, integrated and through multi-disciplinary intervention strategies that include preventive chemotherapy, environmental management, water conservancy, water supply and sanitation development in affected areas and snail control using locally available resources. Such strategies should be evidence-based from research component incorporated in the control activities and use of the most up to date technologies and tools in control. Collaboration would be a platform for capacity strengthening, technology transfer and expertise for the elimination of schistosomiasis from Africa. Above all there is need to obtain government political will for support and sustainability of the programs.

Author details

Takafira Mduluza*, Tawanda J. Chisango, Agness F. Nhidza and Amos Marume

*Address all correspondence to: mduluza@medic.uz.ac.zw

Department of Infection Prevention and Control, School of Laboratory Medicine and Medical Sciences, University of KwaZulu-Natal, Durban, South Africa

References

[1] World Health Organisation, First WHO report on neglected tropical diseases 2010: working to overcome the global impact of neglected tropical diseases. World Health Organisation; Geneva: 2011.

[2] World Health Organization, Preventive chemotherapy in human helminthiasis, coordinated use of anthelminthic drugs in control interventions: a manual for health professionals and programme managers, WHO Press; Geneva, 2006.

[3] WHO, Schistosomiasis fact sheet. World Health Organization; Geneva, Updated February 2016.

[4] Gryseels B, Strickland GM. Schistosomiasis. In: Magill AJ, Hill DR, Solomon T, Ryan ET, editors. Hunter's tropical medicine and emerging infectious disease. 9th ed. Elsevier; Philadelphia, PA, USA: 2013.

[5] Gordon CA, Acosta LP, Gray DJ, Olveda RM, Jarilla B, Gobert GN, Ross AG, McManus DP. High prevalence of *Schistosoma japonicum* infection in Carabao from Samar Province, the Philippines: implications for transmission and control. PLoS Negl Trop Dis. 2012;6(9):e1778. doi:10.1371/journal.pntd.0001778.

[6] He YX, Salafsky B, Ramaswamy K. Comparison of skin invasion among three major species of Schistosoma. Trends Parasitol. 2005;21(5):201–203. Review. PMID: 15837605.

[7] Holick DS, Kaul TL. Schistosomiasis. Urol Nurs. 2013;33(4):163–170.

[8] Chitsulo L, Engels D, Montresor A, Savioli L. The global status of schistosomiasis and its control. Acta Trop. 2000;77(1):41–51. PMID:10996119.

[9] Ekpo UF, Oluwole AS, Abe EM, Etta HE, Olamiju F, Mafiana CF. Schistosomiasis in infants and pre-school-aged children in sub-Saharan Africa: implication for control. Parasitology. 2012;139(7):835–841. doi: 10.1017/S0031182012000029.

[10] Kjetland EF, Poggensee G, Helling-Giese G, Richter J, Sjaastad A, Chitsulo L, Kumwenda N, Gundersen SG, Krantz I, Feldmeier H. Female genital schistosomiasis due to *Schistosoma haematobium*. Clinical and parasitological findings in women in rural Malawi. Acta Trop. 1996;62(4):239–255. PMID: 9028409.

[11] Leutscher PD, Ramarokoto CE, Hoffmann S, Jensen JS, Ramaniraka V, Randrianasolo B, Raharisolo C, Migliani R, Christensen N. Coexistence of urogenital schistosomiasis and sexually transmitted infection in women and men living in an area where *Schistosoma haematobium* is endemic. Clin Infect Dis. 2008;47(6):775–782. doi: 10.1086/591127.

[12] Poggensee G, Kiwelu I, Weger V, Göppner D, Diedrich T, Krantz I, Feldmeier H. Female genital schistosomiasis of the lower genital tract: prevalence and disease-associated morbidity in northern Tanzania. J Infect Dis. 2000;181(3):1210–1213. PMID: 10720558.

[13] Arean VM. Manson's schistosomiasis of the female genital tract. Am J Obstet Gynecol. 1956;72(5):1038–1053. PMID:13362416.

[14] Bullough CH. Infertility and bilharziasis of the female genital tract. Br J Obstet Gynaecol. 1976;83(10):819–822. PMID: 791350.

[15] Okonofua FE, Ojo OS, Odunsi OA, Odesanmi WO. Ectopic pregnancy associated with tubal schistosomiasis in a Nigerian woman. Int J Gynaecol Obstet. 1990;32(3):281–284. PMID:1972123.

[16] Feldmeier H, Krantz I, Poggensee G. Female genital schistosomiasis as a risk-factor for the transmission of HIV. Int J STD AIDS. 1994;5(5):368–372. PMID: 7819359.

[17] Feldmeier H, Krantz I, Poggensee G. Female genital schistosomiasis: a neglected risk factor for the transmission of HIV? Trans R Soc Trop Med Hyg. 1995;89(2):237. PMID: 7778161.

[18] Savioli L, Stansfield S, Bundy DA, Mitchell A, Bhatia R, Engels D, Montresor A, Neira M, Shein AM. Schistosomiasis and soil-transmitted helminth infections: forging control efforts. Trans R Soc Trop Med Hyg. 2002;96(6):577–579. PMID:12625126.

[19] World Health Organization, Report of the WHO informal consultation on the use of praziquantel during pregnancy/lactation and albendazole/mebendazole in children under 24 months. 2003; pp 14–22, WHO, Geneva http://apps.who.int/iris/bitstream/10665/68041/1/WHO_CDS_CPE_PVC_2002.4.pdf.

[20] Mutapi F, Rujeni N, Bourke C, Mitchell K, Appleby L, Nausch N, Midzi N and Mduluza T. Schistosoma haematobium treatment in 1-5 year old children: safety and efficacy of the antihelminthic drug praziquantel. PLoS Negl Trop Dis. 2011;5:e1143. PMID: 21610855.

[21] Crompton DW. The public health importance of hookworm disease. Parasitology. 2000;121(Suppl):S39–S50. PMID: 11386690.

[22] Crompton DW, Whitehead RR. Hookworm infections and human iron metabolism. Parasitology. 1993;107(Suppl):S137–S145. PMID: 8115178.

[23] de Silva NR. Impact of mass chemotherapy on the morbidity due to soil-transmitted nematodes. Acta Trop. 2003;86(2–3):197–214. PMID: 12745137.

[24] Mitchell KM, Mutapi F, Savill NJ, Woolhouse ME. Explaining observed infection and antibody age-profiles in populations with urogenital schistosomiasis. PLoS Comput Biol. 2011;7(10):e1002237. doi: 10.1371/journal.pcbi.1002237. PMID: 22028640.

[25] de Silva NR, Brooker S, Hotez PJ, Montresor A, Engels D, Savioli L. Soil-transmitted helminth infections: updating the global picture. Trends Parasitol. 2003;19(12):547–551. PMID: 14642761.

[26] De Vlas SJ, Engels D, Rabello AL, Oostburg BF, Van Lieshout L, Polderman AM, Van Oortmarssen GJ, Habbema JD, Gryseels B. Validation of a chart to estimate true

Schistosoma mansoni prevalences from simple egg counts. Parasitology. 1997;114 (Pt 2): 113–121. PMID: 9051920.

[27] ten Hove RJ, Verweij JJ, Vereecken K, Polman K, Dieye L, van Lieshout L. Multiplex real-time PCR for the detection and quantificat*ion of Schistosoma mansoni* and *S. haematobium* infection in stool samples collected in northern Senegal. Trans R Soc Trop Med Hyg. 2008;102:179–185. doi: 10.1016/j.trstmh.2007.10.011. PMID: 18177680.

[28] Hamburger J, Hoffman O, Kariuki HC, et al. Large-scale, polymerase chain reaction-based surveillance of *Schistosoma haematobium* DNA in snails from transmission sites in coastal Kenya: a new tool for studying the dynamics of snail infection. Am J Trop Med Hyg. 2004;71:765–773. PMID: 15642969.

[29] Chu KY. Trials of ecological and chemical measures for the control of *Schistosoma haematobium* transmission in a Volta Lake village. Bull World Health Organ. 1978; 56:313–322. PMID: 307458.

[30] Takougang I, Meli J, Wabo Poné J, Angwafo F3rd. Community acceptability of the use of low-dose niclosamide (Bayluscide), as a molluscicide in the control of human schistosomiasis in Sahelian Cameroon. Ann Trop Med Parasitol. 2007;101:479–486. PMID: 17716430.

[31] Mølgaard P, Chihaka A, Lemmich E, Furu P, Windberg C, Ingerslev F, et al. Biodegradability of the molluscicidal saponins of *Phytolacca dodecandra*. Regul Toxicol Pharmacol. 2000;32:248–255. PMID: 11162718.

[32] Ndekha A, Hansen EH, Mølgaard P, Woelk G, Furu P. Community participation as an interactive learning process: experiences from a schistosomiasis control project in Zimbabwe. Acta Trop. 2003;85:325–338. PMID: 12659970.

[33] Evers BN, Madsen H, McKaye KM, Stauffer JR Jr. The schistosome intermediate host, *Bulinus nyassanus*, is a 'preferred' food for the cichlid fish, *Trematocranus placodon*, at Cape Maclear, Lake Malawi. Ann Trop Med Parasitol. 2006;100:75–85. PMID: 16417717 DOI: 10.1179/136485906X78553.

[34] Boelee E, Laamrani H. Environmental control of schistosomiasis through community participation in a Moroccan oasis. Trop Med Int Health. 2004;9:997–1004. PMID: 15361113.

[35] Sleigh A, Li X, Jackson S, Huang K. Eradication of schistosomiasis in Guangxi, China. Part 1: setting, strategies, operations, and outcomes, 1953–92. Bull World Health Organ. 1998;76:361. PMID: 10191554.

[36] Sokhna C, Le Hesran JY, Mbaye PA, Increase of malaria attacks among children presenting concomitant infection by *Schistosoma mansoni* in Senegal. Malar J. 2004;3:43. PMID: 15544703.

[37] Fan KW. Schistosomiasis control and snail elimination in China. Am J Public Health. 2012;102:2231–2232. doi: 10.2105/AJPH.2012.300809. PMID: 23078499.

[38] Pointier JP, Jourdane J. Biological control of the snail hosts of schistosomiasis in areas of low transmission: the example of the Caribbean area. Acta Trop. 2000;77:53–60. PMID: 10996120.

[39] Kloos H. Human behavior, health education and schistosomiasis control: a review. Soc Sci Med. 1995;40: 1497–1511. PMID: 7667655.

[40] Cross RM. Exploring attitudes: the case for Q methodology. Health Educ Res 2005;20: 206–213. PMID: 15385430. DOI: 10.1093/her/cyg121.

[41] Wilson RA, Coulson PS. Immune effector mechanisms against schistosomiasis: looking for a chink in the parasite's armour, Trends Parasitol. 2009;(25):423–431. doi: 10.1016/j.pt.2009.05.011. PMID: 19717340.

[42] Ricciardi A, Ndao M. Still hope for schistosomiasis vaccine. Hum Vaccines Immunother. 2015;(11):2504–2508. doi: 10.1080/21645515.2015.1059981. PMID: 26176659.

[43] Sotillo J, Pearson M, Becker L, Mulvenna J, Loukas A, A quantitative proteomic analysis of the tegumental proteins from Schistosoma mansoni schistosomula reveals novel potential therapeutic targets. Int J Parasitol. 2015;(45):505–516. doi: 10.1016/j.ijpara.2015.03.004. Epub 2015 Apr 21. PMID: 25910674.

[44] Tran MH, Freitas TC, Cooper L, Gaze S, Gatton ML, Jones MK, Lovas E, Pearce EJ, Loukas A. Suppression of mRNAs encoding tegument tetraspanins from Schistosoma mansoni results in impaired tegument turnover. PLoS Pathog. 2010;6(4):e1000840. doi: 10.1371/journal.ppat.1000840. PMID: 20419145.

[45] Molehin AJ, Rojo JU, Siddiqui SZ, Gray SA, Carter D, Siddiqui AA. Development of a schistosomiasis vaccine. Expert Rev Vaccines. 2016;15(5):619–627. PMID: 26651503. DOI: 10.1586/14760584.2016.1131127

[46] Doenhoff MJ, Modha J, Lambertucci JR, McLaren DJ. The immune dependence of chemotherapy. Parasitol Today. 1991;7:16–18. PMID: 15463377.

[47] Wilson RA. The saga of schistosome migration and attrition. Parasitology. 2009;136:1581–1592. doi: 10.1017/S0031182009005708. PMID: 19265564.

[48] Warren KS. Regulation of the prevalence and intensity of schistosomiasis in man: immunology or ecology? J Infect Dis. 1973;127:595–609. PMID: 4572813.

[49] Kjetland EF, Ndhlovu PD, Gomo E, Mduluza T, Midzi N, Gwanzura L, Mason PR, Sandvik L, Friis H, Gundersen SG. Association between genital schistosomiasis and HIV in rural Zimbabwean women. AIDS. 2006;20(4):593–600. PMID: 16470124.

[50] Reimert CM, Fitzsimmons CM, Joseph S, Mwatha JK, Jones FM, Kimani G, Hoffmann KF, Booth M, Kabatereine NB, Dunne DW, Vennervald BJ. Eosinophil activity in Schistosoma mansoni infections in vivo and in vitro in relation to plasma cytokine profile pre- and posttreatment with praziquantel. Clin Vaccine Immunol. 2006;13(5): 584–593. PMID:16682480.

[51] Fitzsimmons CM, Jones FM, Pinot de Moira A, Protasio AV, Khalife J, Dickinson HA, Tukahebwa EM, Dunne DW. Progressive cross-reactivity in IgE responses: an explanation for the slow development of human immunity to schistosomiasis? Infect Immun. 2012;80(12):4264-4270. doi: 10.1128/IAI.00641-12. PMID: 23006852.

[52] Nausch N, Louis D, Lantz O, Peguillet I, Trottein F, Chen IY, Appleby LJ, Bourke CD, Midzi N, Mduluza T, Mutapi F. Age-related patterns in human myeloid dendritic cell populations in people exposed to Schistosoma haematobium infection. PLoS Negl Trop Dis. 2012;6(9):e1824. doi: 10.1371/journal.pntd.0001824. PMID: 23029585.

[53] Lyke KE, Dicko A, Dabo A, Sangare L, Kone A, Coulibaly D, Guindo A, Traore K, Daou M, Diarra I, Sztein MB, Plowe CV, Doumbo OK. Association of *Schistosoma haematobium* infection with protection against acute *Plasmodium falciparum* malaria in Malian children. Am J Trop Med Hyg. 2005;73(6):1124–1130. PMID:16354824.

[54] Briand V, Watier L, LE Hesran JY, Garcia A, Cot M. Coinfection with *Plasmodium falciparum* and *Schistosoma haematobium*: protective effect of schistosomiasis on malaria in Senegalese children? Am J Trop Med Hyg. 2005;72:702–707. PMID: 13964953.

[55] Abel L, Marquet S, Chevillard C, elWali NE, Hillaire D, Dessein A. Genetic predisposition to bilharziasis in humans: research methods and application to the study of Schistosoma mansoni infection, J Soc Biol. 2000;194(1):15–18. PMID: 11107544.

[56] Kouriba B, Chevillard C, Bream JH, Argiro L, Dessein H, Arnaud V, Sangare L, Dabo A, Beavogui AH, Arama C, Traoré HA, Doumbo O, Dessein A. Analysis of the 5q31-q33 locus shows an association between IL13-1055C/T IL-13-591A/G polymorphisms and *Schistosoma haematobium* infections. J Immunol. 2005;174(10):6274–6281. PMID: 15879126.

[57] Mduluza T, Gori E, Chitongo P, Midzi N, Ruwona T, Soko W, Mlambo G, Mutambu SL, Kumar N. Analysis of TNF-α and IL-10 gene polymorphisms in Zimbabwean children exposed to malaria. Afr J Biotechnol. 2013;1034–1039. DOI: 10.5897/AJB12.2443

[58] Bendtzen K. Natural and therapy-induced antibodies to cytokines. Drug Discov Today. 2004;9(6):259. PMID: 15003242.

[59] Jia T-W, Melville S, Utzinger J, King CH, Zhou XN. Soil-transmitted helminth reinfection after drug treatment: a systematic review and meta-analysis. PLoS Negl Trop Dis. 2010;6(5): e1621. doi:10.1371/journal.pntd.0001621.

[60] Anderson R, Truscott J, Hollingsworth TD. The coverage and frequency of mass drug administration required to eliminate persistent transmission of soil-transmitted helminths. Phil Trans R Soc. 2014;B 369: 20130435. http://dx.doi.org/10.1098/rstb.2013.0435.

[61] Sesay S, Paye J, Bah MS, McCarthy FM, Conteh A, Sonnie M, Hodges MH, Zhang Y. Schistosoma mansoni infection after three years of mass drug administration in Sierra Leone. Parasit Vectors. 2014 ;7:14. doi: 10.1186/1756-3305-7-14. PMID: 24401567.

[62] Anderson RM, Turner HC, Farrell SH, Yang J, Truscott JE. What is required in terms of mass drug administration to interrupt the transmission of schistosome parasites in regions of endemic infection? Parasit Vectors. 2015;8:553. doi: 10.1186/s13071-015-1157-y. PMID: 26489831.

[63] Hodges MH, Dada N, Warmsley A, Paye J, Bangura MM, Nyorkor E, Sonnie M, Zhang Y. Mass drug administration significantly reduces infection of *Schistosoma mansoni* and hookworm in school children in the national control program in Sierra Leone. BMC Infect Dis. 2012;12:16. doi: 10.1186/1471-2334-12-16. PMID: 22264258.

[64] Chami GF, Kontoleon AA, Bulte E, Fenwick A, Kabatereine NB, Tukahebwa EM, Dunne DW. Profiling nonrecipients of mass drug administration for schistosomiasis and hookworm infections: a comprehensive analysis of praziquantel and albendazole coverage in community-directed treatment in Uganda. Clin Infect Dis. 2016;62(2): 200–207. doi: 10.1093/cid/civ829.

[65] Araujo N, Mattos AC, Coelho PM, Katz N. Association of oxamniquine praziquantel and clonazepam in experimental *Schistosomiasis mansoni*. Mem Inst Oswaldo Cruz. 2008;103(8):781–785. PMID: 19148417.

[66] Ferrari MLA, Coelho PMZ, Antunes CMF, Tavares CAP, da Cunha AS. Efficacy of oxamniquine and praziquantel in the treatment of Schistosoma mansoni infection: a controlled trial. Bull World Health Organ. 2003;81(3):190–196. PMID: 12764515. PMCID: PMC2572425.

[67] Cupit PM, Cunningham C. What is the mechanism of action of praziquantel and how might resistance strike? Future Med Chem. 2015;7(6):701–705. doi: 10.4155/fmc.15.11.

[68] Doenhoff MJ, Cioli D, Utzinger J. Praziquantel: mechanisms of action, resistance and new derivatives for schistosomiasis. Curr Opin Infect Dis. 2008;21(6):659–667. doi: 10.1097/QCO.0b013e328318978f. PMID:18978535.

[69] Alvela-Suárez L, Velasco-Tirado V, Belhassen-Garcia M, Novo-Veleiro I, Pardo-Lledías J, Romero-Alegría A, Pérez del Villar L, Valverde-Merino MP, Cordero-Sánchez M. Safety of the combined use of praziquantel and albendazole in the treatment of human hydatid disease. Am J Trop Med Hyg. 2014; 90(5):819–822. doi: 10.4269/ajtmh.13-0059. PMID: 24615131.

[70] King CH, Muchiri EM, Ouma JH. Evidence against rapid emergence of praziquantel resistance in *Schistosoma haematobium*, Kenya. Emerg Infect Dis. 2000;6(6):585–594. PMID:11076716.

[71] Rujeni N, Nausch N, Midzi N, Cowan GJ, Burchmore R, Cavanagh DR, Taylor DW, Mduluza T, Mutapi F. Immunological consequences of antihelminthic treatment in preschool children exposed to urogenital schistosome infection. J Trop Med. 2013;2013:283619. doi: 10.1155/2013/283619.

[72] Midzi N, Mduluza T, Chimbari MJ, Tshuma C, Charimari L, Mhlanga G, Manangazira P, Munyati SM, Phiri I, Mutambu SL, Midzi SS, Ncube A, Muranzi

LP, Rusakaniko S, Mutapi F. Distribution of schistosomiasis and soil transmitted helminthiasis in Zimbabwe: towards a national plan of action for control and elimination. PLoS Negl Trop Dis. 2014;8(8):e3014. doi: 10.1371/journal.pntd.0003014. PMID: 25121489.

[73] Zhou XN, Xu J, Chen HG, Wang TP, Huang XB, Lin DD, Wang QZ, Tang L, Guo JG, Wu XH, Feng T, Chen JX, Guo J, Chen SH, Li H, Wu ZD, Peeling RW. Tools to support policy decisions related to treatment strategies and surveillance of *Schistosomiasis japonica* towards elimination. PLoS Negl Trop Dis. 2011;5(12):e1408. doi: 10.1371/journal.pntd.0001408. PMID: 22206024.